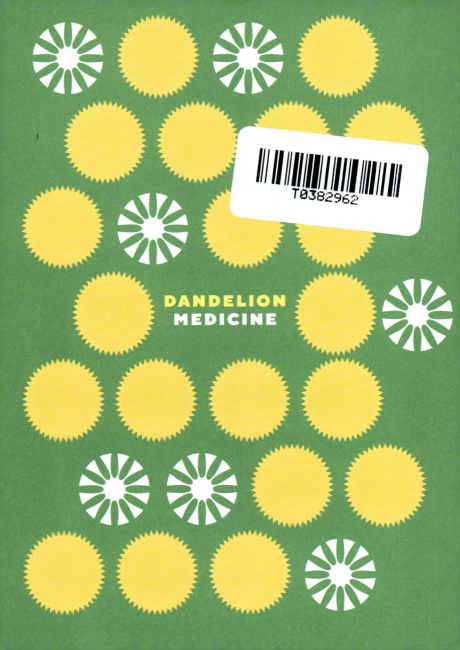

DANDELION
MEDICINE

T0382962

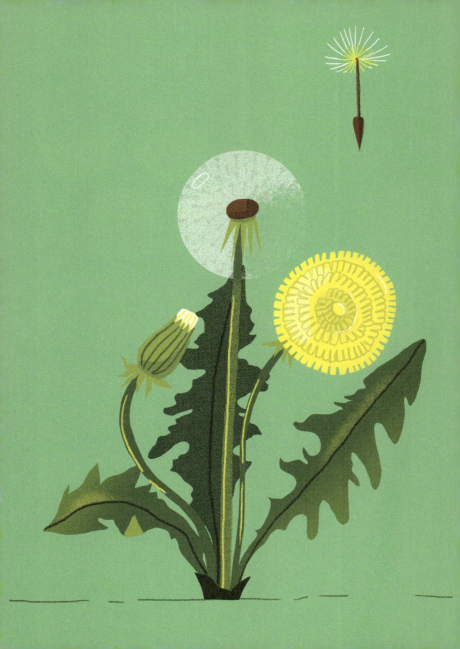

DANDELION MEDICINE

FORAGE, FEAST, AND NOURISH YOURSELF
with This Extraordinary Weed

BRIGITTE MARS

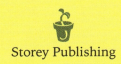

Storey Publishing

*The mission of Storey Publishing is to serve our customers by
publishing practical information that encourages
personal independence in harmony with the environment.*

Edited by Carleen Madigan
Art direction and book design by Carolyn Eckert
Text production by Jennifer Jepson Smith

Cover illustrations by © Michelle Delabre, except
back (b.) by Britton, N.L., and A. Brown, 1913,
*An illustrated flora of the northern United States,
Canada and the British Possessions.* 3 vols.
Provided by Kentucky Native Plant Society, NY/
USDA-NRCS PLANTS Database

Interior illustrations by © Alina Tyshchuk, 41;
Alison Kolesar © Storey Publishing, LLC, 53, 91,
123; © Beth Walrond, 2; Beverly Duncan © Storey
Publishing, LLC, 88 t., 92, 95–97, 100–103, 106; de
Boodt, Anselmus Boëtius/Rijksmuseum/CC0 1.0/
Wikimedia Commons/public domain, 121 t.; The
British Library/Flickr Commons/Wikimedia, 14;
Britton, N.L., and A. Brown, 1913, *An illustrated
flora of the northern United States, Canada and the
British Possessions.* 3 vols. Provided by Kentucky
Native Plant Society, NY/USDA-NRCS PLANTS
Database, 21, 26, 58 b., 107; Bunchō, Tani/The
Yale University Art Gallery/CC0 1.0, 34; Carolyn
Eckert © Storey Publishing, LLC, 15, 26, 58 t., 86,
184; © Ceri Lineham, 133; Charles Joslin
© Storey Publishing, LLC, 88 b., 94 t.; © Christopher
Dina, 72; © Clairice Gifford, 8; Codex/Wikimedia
Commons/CC BY-SA 3.0, 63; Dorothy P. Lathrop,
Down-Adown-Derry/public domain, 23; Ewing,
Juliana Horatia, "Old Father Christmas and Other
Tales," illustrated by Gordon Brownie and Other
Artists/Wikimedia/public domain, 61; © Flo Rees,
117; Hamilton, Edward, *Leotodon Taraxacum*
Plate 62 from *Flora Homoeopathica* by Edward
Hamilton/Wikimedia Commons/public domain, 28
t.l., 29 b.l. & b.r.; © Kristen Drozdowski, 5; © Laura
Velasco/@diablo_puerco, 67; Lindman, C. A. M.
(Carl Axel Magnus), *Billeder af Nordens Flora*/Flickr
Commons/Wikimedia, 28 b.r., 29 t.r. & t.l., 185;
© Liv Lee, 138; Mansfield, Ira Franklin, Contributions
to the flora of Beaver County, from the Mansfield
Herbarium, 1865–1903/Internet Archive Book
Images/FlickrCommons/Wikimedia/public domain,
60; Müller, Walther Otto, from *Köhler's Medizinal-
Pflanzen*/Wikimedia Commons/public domain,
13, 28 t.r. & b.l.; Photograph © 2023 Museum of
Fine Arts, Boston, 25; © Owen Davey, 43; Pieper,
Charles J., Wilbur L. Beauchamp, and Orlin D. Frank.
Everyday Problems in Biology (W. J. Gage and
Company, 1939)/Open Library, 45; Randy Mosher
© Storey Publishing, LLC, 85; Regina Hughes ©
Storey Publishing, LLC, 19; © Salli S. Swindell, 38;
© Sally Caulwell, 75; © Sarah Abbott, 46, 49, 135;
Sarah Brill © Storey Publishing, LLC, 44, 51, 89, 93,
94 b., 98, 99, 108, 121 b., 137, 163; © Theo Dagadita/
ephemre, 55; Vitus Auslasser/Wikimedia Commons/
Public domain, 192; © Yoko Isami, 111

Text © 1999, 2023 by Brigitte Mars

This publication is intended to provide educational
information for the reader on the covered subject.
It is not intended to take the place of personalized
medical counseling, diagnosis, and treatment from
a trained health professional. Please consult a
physician or other health professional if needed.

Storey books are available at special discounts
when purchased in bulk for premiums and sales
promotions as well as for fund-raising or educational
use. Special editions or book excerpts can also be
created to specification. For details, please send an
email to special.markets@hbgusa.com.

Storey Publishing
210 MASS MoCA Way
North Adams, MA 01247
storey.com

Storey Publishing is an imprint of Workman
Publishing, a division of Hachette Book Group, Inc.,
1290 Avenue of the Americas, New York, NY 10104.
The Storey Publishing name and logo are registered
trademarks of Hachette Book Group, Inc.

ISBNs: 978-1-63586-763-3 (paperback);
978-1-63586-764-0 (ebook)

Printed in the United States by Versa (interior) and
PC (cover) on paper from responsible sources
10 9 8 7 6 5 4 3

Library of Congress Cataloging-in-Publication Data
on file

For my beloved daughters,
Sunflower Sparkle Mars and Rainbeau Harmony Mars,
and their children,
Jade Destiny Mars, Solwyn Forest Stegall,
and Luna Zara Mars

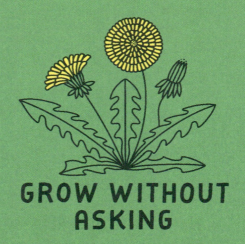

GROW WITHOUT
ASKING

CONTENTS

1

2

3

4

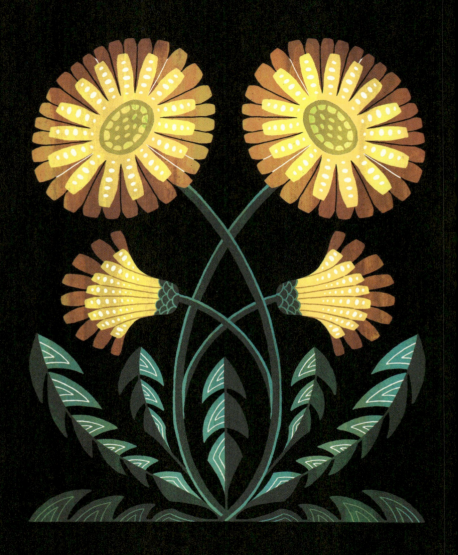

Dandelion!

Don't you be cryin'

We're doing our best to tell the world about you!

Sunshine bright

You ray of light

Concentrating solar energy

You are free

Growing all around me

Blessed be

Yeah God!

Ray of gold

I am told

Helps heal people and the planet

I do believe

It is time to perceive

The truth about weeds

That fulfill so many of our needs

Breathe deep the breath of life!

Hurrah, Dandy Lion!

—*Brigitte Mars*

CHAPTER
1

THE VIRTUES
of the
DANDELION

The dandelion may well be the world's most famous weed. It has been said that the average American recognizes more than a thousand logos for commercial products yet recognizes fewer than five plants that grow in his or her area. For most people, the dandelion is likely to be one of these familiar plants—though it's *un*likely that those people know its benefits. As Ralph Waldo Emerson wrote, "What is a weed? A plant whose virtues have not yet been discovered." The time has come again to learn the virtues of the dandelion.

Meet the Dandelion!

Each spring, dandelions burst into a carpet of sunny yellow blossoms, creating a cheerful addition to the landscape after a long winter. The flowers open wide to greet the morning and offer nectar for pollinators, then close toward evening. Though the dandelion is considered by many people to be a useless weed, in truth it is one of the most beneficial and healthful of herbs.

Every part of the dandelion has a use, ranging from food to medicine to dye. These beneficial properties did not always go unnoticed in North America; up until the 1800s, people would actually pull the grass out of their yards to make room for dandelions and other useful "weeds" such as chickweed, mallow, and chamomile.

Botanical Origins

The botanical name for dandelion is *Taraxacum officinale*. The genus name, *Taraxacum*, is from Arabic and means "bitter herb." It may have evolved from the Greek *taraxos*, a term used by Arab physicians of the early Middle Ages to mean "disorder," and *akos*, meaning "remedy." Or it could be derived from the Greek *taraxia*, meaning "eye disorder," and *akeomai*, "to cure," as dandelion was traditionally used as a remedy for the eyes.

The species name, *officinale*, tells us that the plant is or was an "official medicine" or "the plant of the apothecaries in Rome."

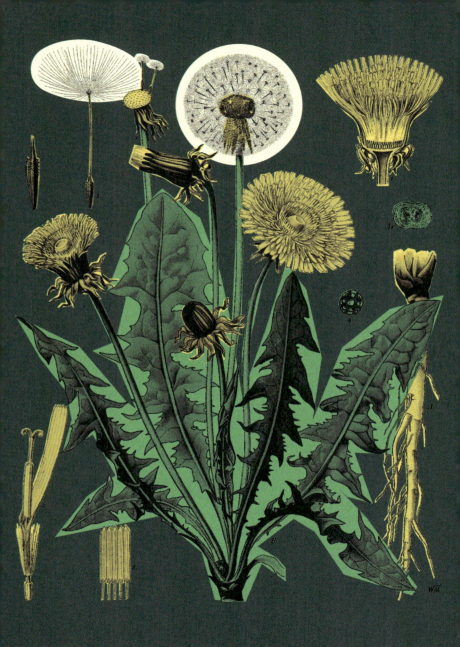

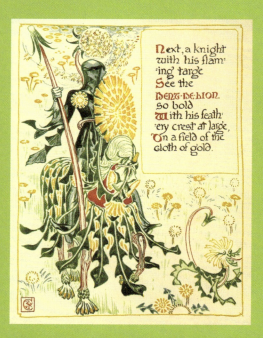

Next, a knight
with his flam-
ing targe
See the
DENT-DE-LION,
so bold
With his feath-
ery crest at large,
On a field of the
cloth of gold.

What's in a Name?

**Opinions differ on the origin of dandelion's genus name,
Taraxacum. Some believe that it derives from the Persian
talkh chakok, "bitter herb." The common name dandelion
derives from the French *dent-de-lion*, "tooth of the lion,"
in reference to the jagged shape of the leaves.**

**Each of the florets has five toothed edges, another
correlation to lion's teeth. Some say the comparison to
lions has to do with the flower's bright yellow color; others
say simply that the plant is as strong as the tooth of a lion.
The name may also symbolize the traditional astrological
connection between the sun and lions—Leo (the Lion)
is governed by the Sun.**

A Dandelion by Any Other Name

Around the world, the dandelion is well known and named:

Chinese: *chian-nou-ts'ao, huang-hua ti-ting*

French: *piss-en-lit, dent-de-lion* German: *Wenzahn, Kuhblume, Löwenzahn*

Greek: *radiki*
(meaning "radiating from the center")

Hindi: *dudhal* Icelandic: *túnfill*

Italian: *dente di leone, tarasso, soffione* Japanese: *hokoei*

Korean: *p'ogongyong* Mandarin: *pú gong ying*

Persian: *talkh chakok* ("bitter herb") Russian: *oduvanchik, pushki*

Sanskrit: *dughdapheni* Spanish: *diente de león*

Turkish: *kara hindiba otu, yabani* Welsh: *dant y llew*

DANDY NICKNAMES

Dandelion has also been known by a variety of nicknames, including:

amarga

bitterwort

blowball

cankerwort

chicoria

clockflower

consuelda

devil's milkpail

doonhead clock

fairy clock

fortune-teller

heart-fever grass

Irish daisy

milk gowan

milk witch

monk's head

peasant's cloak

puffball

priest's crown

sun in the grass

swine's snout

tell-time

tramp with the golden head

piss-en-lit*

piddly bed

wet-a-bed

wild endive

yellow gowan

* meaning "pee in the bed"

Each of the names has historical or cultural significance.
For example, *gowan* is a Scottish word for
"daisylike flower."

Names such as **blowball** and **tell-time** are reminders of a **traditional game:**
Children blow the seed heads
and watch them disperse and fly away;
the number left is supposed to signify the hour.

When the mature flower head closes,
it resembles a **pig's snout**;
hence the nickname **swine's snout**.

The plant is sometimes known as
monk's head—when all the seeds have gone,
the top looks like a **priest's tonsure**,
or shaved crown.

Botanical Features

Dandelion is believed to be native to Greece and the Mediterranean regions of Asia Minor and Europe. It is a perennial member of the Asteraceae family, which is one of the largest groups of flowering plants and includes daisies, sunflowers, and calendula as well as Jerusalem artichokes, lettuce, and endive.

Leaves

Dandelion is considered by botanists to be a dicot—that is, a plant that bears two leaves from its germinating seed. The hollow, unbranched stems grow 2 to 18 inches high atop a rosette of shiny, hairless, coarsely toothed green leaves that are broader toward the top than at the base. The teeth of the leaves are usually directed downward. The leaves grow in a basal rosette—quite an ingenious botanical design, as the natural grooving of the leaves helps to steer water to the roots of the plant.

Flowers

The plant first blooms, one yellow flower head per plant, in early spring. The blossom, measuring ½ to 2 inches in diameter, is actually a compilation of about 150 florets, each a complete tiny tube-shaped ray flower in its own right with anthers and stigmas. Each floret has five tiny teeth on its edge.

The flowering season in the Northern Hemisphere, where dandelions are most common, is from April to June. The blossoms close early in the evening and during cloudy weather, perhaps to protect the nectar and pollen as well as to conserve heat during cold spring nights. Dandelions are very sensitive to temperature; they bloom more when the weather is cool and

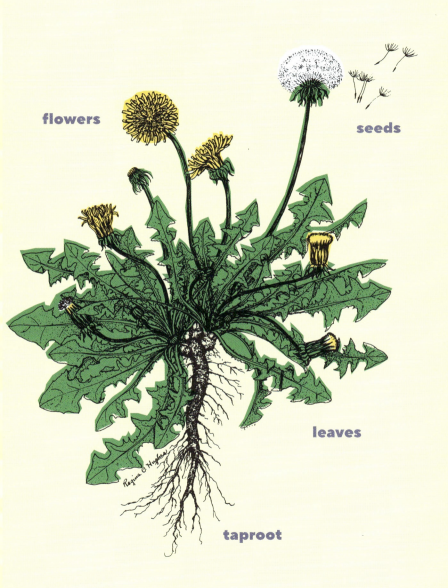

flowers

seeds

leaves

taproot

The seeds, borne on a circular ball, are known as acheniums. They ... are carried on the wind— often as many as 5 miles from their origin.

clear and disappear as hot summer arrives. Dandelion has one of the longest flowering seasons of any plant, and when a warm spell occurs in an off-season, it is not unusual to see the pretty yellow flowers. A second flowering may occur in fall from seeds that self-sowed earlier in the growing season.

Underneath the flower is a green calyx with downward-curved outer bracts. When the blossoming cycle is complete, the flower head folds up for several days, with the calyx drawn into a cylindrical shape around the ripening ovaries, before reopening to reveal its parachute-topped seeds. Dandelion is considered apomict: It produces seeds without pollination or fertilization. This asexual tendency enables many forms of the plant to evolve, each differing from another in minute ways. The seeds, borne on a circular ball, are known as acheniums. They bear a feathery pappus (or tuft) and are carried on the wind—often as many as 5 miles from their origin. The ovule contains special cells that produce embryos identical to the parent plant.

Root

The long taproot issues from a short rhizome. All of the underground portions are dark brown on the outside, milky white on the inside. The taproot can grow up to a foot long, which allows the plant access to water deep in the earth so that it can survive dry spells. The entire plant contains a milky white juice.

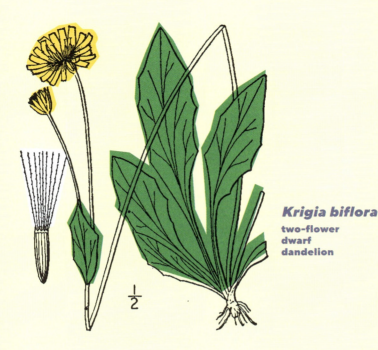

Krigia biflora
two-flower
dwarf
dandelion

$\frac{1}{2}$

Related Species

There are more than 250 useful species related to dandelion,
Taraxacum erythrospermum (red-seeded dandelion),
T. ceratophorum (horned dandelion), *T. lyratum* (alpine dandelion),
Leontodon autumnalis (fall dandelion or hawkbit), and
Krigia virginica (dwarf dandelion). To identify a dandelion cousin,
remember that dandelions grow with an unbranching
stem from a rosette of leaves. Any plant that has branching
characteristics is not a dandelion relation.

Lore and Legend

Because dandelions can be found in many parts of the world, there are many different legends and folkloric stories explaining how the dandelion came to be. Dandelions also predominate in the traditional mythology of many cultures. For example, ancient Greek mythology tells the tale of Hecate, goddess of the earth and underworld, honoring Theseus with a salad of dandelion greens after he slew the infamous Minotaur.

Fairies and Wood Sprites

Following in the footsteps of many other creation stories, one popular legend ascribes dandelion's birth to the work of fairies. Many thousands of years ago, when the world was populated with fairies and elves, the first humans arrived. They soon caused these tiny creatures many problems, as the humans were usually unable to see the wee folk and would step on them. So the fairies took to dressing in bright yellow garments and eventually were changed into dandelions, which have the ability to spring back up if trodden upon. Thus, it is believed that dandelions recover so quickly from being stepped on because each contains the spirit of a fairy.

Another folk story tells of a miserly old man who discovered a pot of gold at the end of a rainbow. He decided to hide it in the ground rather than share his good fortune. In order to think about where he would bury it, he took the gold home with him in a sack and then went to bed. While he was sleeping, a hungry mouse, in search of food, gnawed a hole in the sack.

Early the next morning, the man grabbed the sack and went to bury it. As he reached a dark part of the forest, he noticed how light the sack had become. When he looked inside,

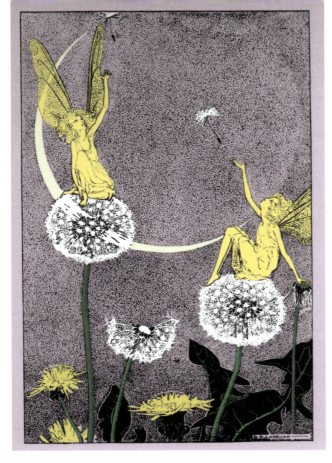

there were but a few coins left. "My gold has fallen out!" he cried. "I shall retrace my steps and pick it all back up!" Believing the nuggets would be easy to spot on the ground, he walked back and bent down to collect the shiny gold pieces. However, they had become rooted to the ground. When he looked closer, he noticed that each coin was now a golden flower. Wood sprites had transformed the coins into golden flowers for all to enjoy.

Native American Stories

An Ojibwe legend holds that a beautiful, golden-haired maiden was once admired by the South Wind. The South Wind was too lazy to court her, so he lay in the shade and watched her as she smelled the flowers. He waited so long that one day, when awakening from a nap, he noticed that she was now a gray-haired woman. The South Wind blamed his brother the North Wind, believing it was he who had blown a frost upon her to whiten her golden hair. To this day, the South Wind continues to sigh for the love he may have once enjoyed.

Another Indigenous legend involves a golden-haired girl who fell in love with the Sun. She rejected all suitors and simply watched the Sun make his journey across the sky, although he ignored her. She grieved until she got old, frail, and gray and was blown away by the wind. The Sun, finally noticing, felt sorry that he had not paid attention to her and could not bring her back. The Great Spirit took pity and sent small golden flowers to bloom on the prairies, and to this day the wind carries off the gray-haired seeds.

The Doctrine of Signatures

The doctrine of signatures is an ancient belief system stating that a plant's appearance hints at what part of the body it can treat. The concept evolved from bits of astrology, alchemy, fact, and fantasy. The doctrine is founded on the belief that by observing a plant—the color of its flower, the shape of its leaf or root—you can determine its place in nature's plan. For example, the form of kidney beans tells us that they're good for the kidneys; blood-red beets fortify the blood; a head of cauliflower benefits the brain.

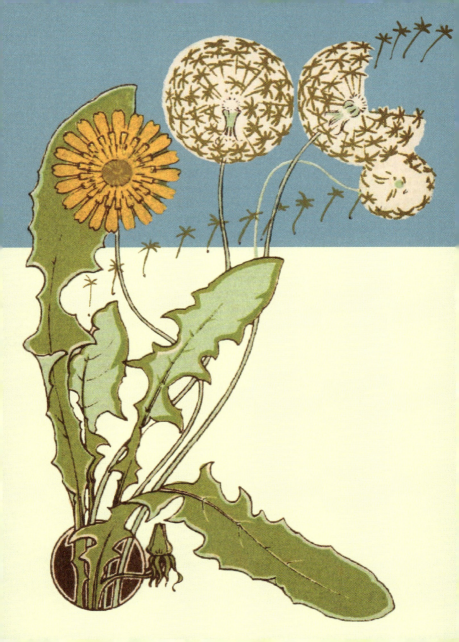

magic and mystery

In the sixteenth century, Pietro Andrea Mattioli, an Italian physician and author of *Commentarii in sex libros Pedacii Dioscorides Anazarbei de medica materia*, wrote, "Magicians say that if a person rubs himself all over with dandelion, he will be everywhere welcome and obtain what he wishes." Rubbing your skin with dandelion juice was believed to ensure you would receive hospitality in any home.

According to astrology, dandelion corresponds to the air element. It is governed by Jupiter and considered a masculine plant. Herbs ruled by Jupiter are cheerful, benevolent, soothing, and jovial. Dandelion is also under the dominion of the Sun, which governs plants of a bright golden color. In Ayurvedic medicine, however, dandelion is ruled by Saturn, which governs cool, bitter, and detoxifying herbs.

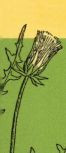

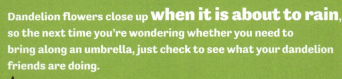

Dandelion flowers close up **when it is about to rain**, so the next time you're wondering whether you need to bring along an umbrella, just check to see what your dandelion friends are doing.

What Dandelion Tells Us

Dandelion is a survivor. It reaches deep into the earth, making it impervious to burrowing animals and fire. The bright yellow color of the flower corresponds to the liver, according to the principles of traditional Chinese medicine, and thus explains its use in treating gallstones and jaundice. Because dandelion has a juicy stem and root, the doctrine of signatures indicated that it was beneficial for increasing urine production. The roots and leaves are associated with the physical body, the yellow flowers with mental health, and the puffball seed head with emotional well-being. As the seeds fly off and return to the earth, they represent the muscular structure being calmed.

Dandelion is considered a supreme remedy for liver health. The liver is an organ that has suffered numerous assaults from chemicals in our environment. So, too, has the dandelion—yet it continues to adapt, and helps the human organism adapt, as well. Dandelion is indeed hardy. It grows through cracks in sidewalks; thrives despite a multitude of herbicides; and can even withstand 20,000 volts of electricity. Where lawns are mowed, the dandelion keeps a very short stem, but in tall grass the stems stretch to greater height to catch the rays of the sun. If the leaves or flowers are cut, more grow back within a few days. It seems fitting that a plant that has adjusted so well to the environment can help humans adapt to a polluted planet—while we do our best to correct the situation. The simple abundance of the dandelion may perhaps be a sign that we should be using lots of this gift of nature!

Other Folklore Beliefs

There are so many wonderful facts and so many myths about this plant! Following are just a few bits of dandelion lore that have been passed down to me.

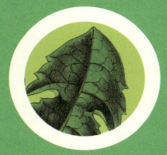

Drinking a tea of dandelion leaves is said to promote psychic ability, especially if you drink the tea while visualizing an increase in that talent.

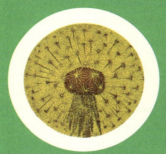

Maidens would blow on the seed head; the number of seeds remaining would determine how many children they would have once married.

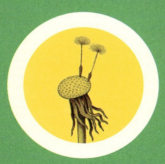

When a maiden blew on a dandelion seed head, if at least one seed remained, it was a sign that her sweetheart was thinking of her.

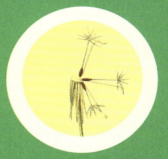

When the downy seeds blow off the dandelion and there is no wind, it will rain.

In the Victorian language of flowers, dandelion signifies love. It is also a symbol of wishes, welcome, faithfulness, and divination. In some cultures, it is considered good luck to dream of dandelions; in others, though, a dandelion dream portends ill fortune, indicating that the dreamer's lover was untrue.

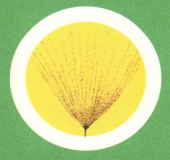

Lovers should blow dandelion seeds in the direction of their beloved to send messages of affection.

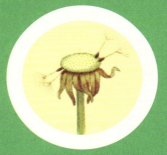

Blow on a dandelion seed head, and however many seeds are left are how many more years you will live.

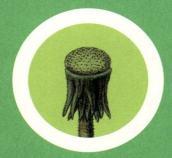

Make a wish, then blow on the seed head. If every single seed flies away, your wish will come true.

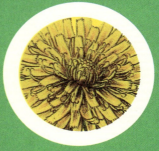

Growing dandelions at the northwest corner of your property is said to bring favorable winds.

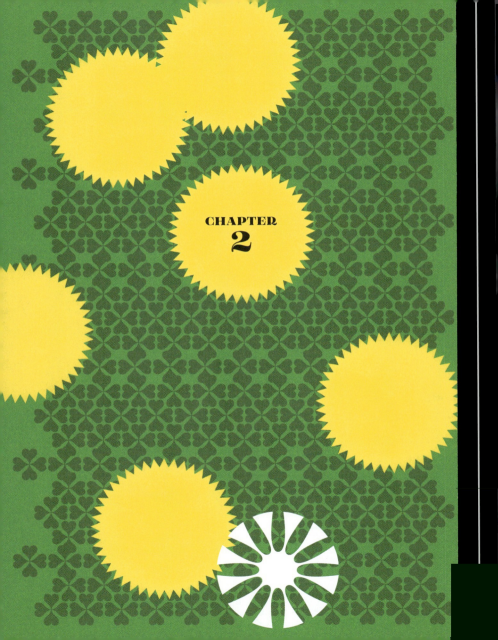

CHAPTER
2

Collecting, Growing, and HARVESTING

Dandelions grow worldwide except in deserts and in the tropics. This herb seems to follow the steps of civilization and cultivation; it is especially prolific throughout the northern temperate zones and can flourish from sea level up to altitudes of 10,500 feet. There are even reports of a variety growing in the Himalayas at 18,000 feet!

Benefits for the Soil and the Environment

Dandelion grows where the soil is healthy—it is considered an indicator of the presence of potassium, magnesium, calcium, and sodium. Dandelions prefer loose, rich, well-drained soil with neutral acidity, but they can tolerate a wide range of conditions. Because of dandelion's deep taproot, it doesn't compete with short-rooted grasses. The long roots aerate the soil, providing drainage channels for water, and help heal barren or overworked soil by soaking up nutrients that have been washed downward and bringing them up toward the surface where other, shorter-rooted plants can use them—sort of like an herbal earthworm: facilitating, not competing. Dandelions also work in symbiosis with bacteria to pull nitrogen from the air and convert it to nitrates in the soil. They are natural soil enhancers, as earthworms enjoy the soil near them (hence the Chinese nickname "earth nail").

Dandelions growing in fruit orchards give off ethylene gas at sunset, which helps fruit ripen early and evenly. Not only do the fruits grow larger, but so, too, do the dandelions. They seem to have a cooperative, symbiotic relationship.

When dandelions die, the channels formed by their roots open up the earth for other plants to grow. If uprooted dandelions are added to compost, they work as an activator, speeding up the decomposition of composted material and making copper available as a nutrient.

Where the dandelion grows, the garden will flourish. —*old farmers' saying*

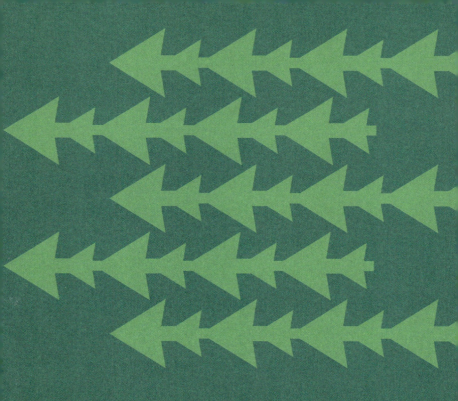

Surviving on Dandelion

Should you find yourself in a survival situation with nothing to eat except old dandelion greens, boil the leaves in two changes of water to remove the bitter flavor. The plant has even been used as survival food in polar regions.

Boy Scouts learn that the seedlike fruits (found on the stem, at the base of the "parachute"), though somewhat bitter, can be eaten raw in an emergency—remove the plumelike hairs by rubbing the seeds in your palms to separate them from the stalks.

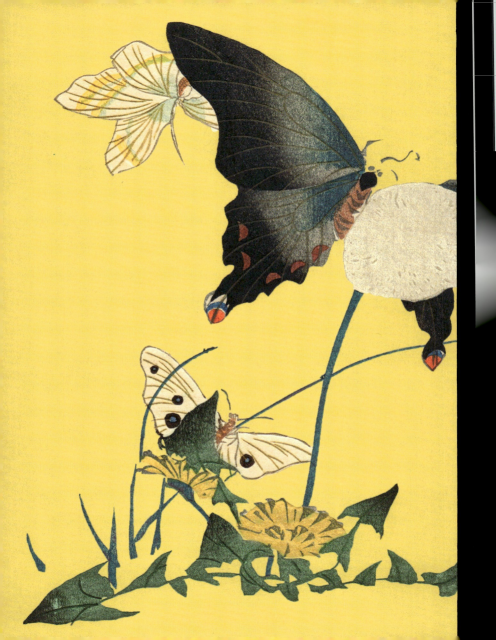

A Friend to Creatures

Dandelion blooms in early spring when other sources of pollen are scarce. The stigma of the flower grows through the tube formed from the anthers. The stigma pushes the pollen forward, which coats visiting insects who then carry it to other flowers and thus ensure cross-pollination. It has been reported that at least 85 different insects are nourished by dandelions, including butterflies, wasps, flies, and beetles. Bees love it—dandelion is an important plant for honey production.

Grouse, pheasants, Canada geese, and many other birds eat the seeds. Purple finches are particularly attracted to dandelions. The leaves are consumed by black bears and grizzly bears, chipmunks, elk, and porcupines. Goats, pigs, and rabbits will eat the whole plant. You can feed dandelions to domestic rabbits, guinea pigs, and gerbils. Cows may not relish the bitter flavor of dandelion, but when they eat it they produce even more milk. Dandelions are a favorite food for chickens. Horses will eat dandelion greens and roots when they are cut and mixed with bran. The leaves are fed to silkworms when their usual food, mulberry leaves, is scarce.

Growing Habits

Dandelions are abundant in meadows, in waste places, along roadsides, and, of course, in lawns. The plant frequently grows where the soil has been disturbed. You'll often find dandelion as a companion to plantain, clover, and alfalfa.

Dandelion leaves lie flat, so the plant usually remains unharmed by the lawnmower. If you try to dig it up and inadvertently leave just a small portion of the root in the soil,

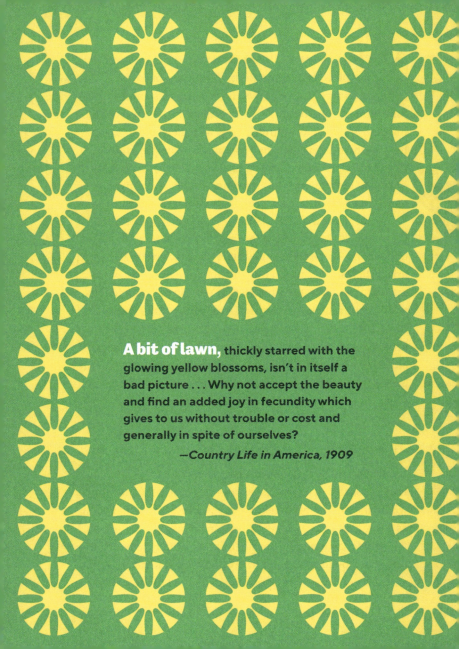

A bit of lawn, thickly starred with the glowing yellow blossoms, isn't in itself a bad picture . . . Why not accept the beauty and find an added joy in fecundity which gives to us without trouble or cost and generally in spite of ourselves?

—*Country Life in America, 1909*

another plant will emerge. While many plant species are being lost to industrialization and the building of housing developments and shopping centers where once there were meadows, dandelion has shown a remarkable ability to adapt to environmental stress; it thrives in disturbed or compacted soils and near roads and highways. It will even sprout up through the cracks in your sidewalk. I believe it wants to be here!

Dandelion has many physical traits that enhance its ability to proliferate. Flowers form at the top of the root long before the final frost of winter, giving them the protection of several inches of soil and ensuring a long blooming season. The seeds are a type of flying apparatus with radiating threads that form a sort of parachute. When wind sweeps across, the seeds are, in the words of David Attenborough in *The Private Life of Plants*, like a "fragile elegant globe. Even the gentlest breath, from the wind or a child, can cause squadrons to take off and sail high and far through the sky." Seeds have been found as far away as 5 miles from their mother plant. Also, the seeds do not have to go through a long germination period, and thus they need less time to grow than do many other plants.

Cultivating Your Own

French seed catalogs from the late 1800s and early 1900s offered as many as five different varieties of dandelion. Given the plant's versatility, it's not surprising that dandelion is cultivated and sold in marketplaces in many parts of the world. We in North America are just catching on. Today, dandelion seeds are commercially available from many seed catalogs. Or you can collect seed from the wild. To do so, cover the flowering

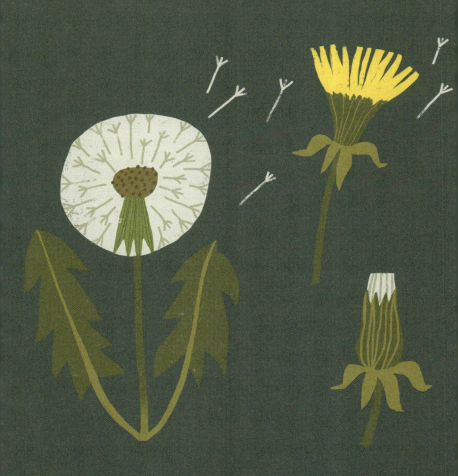

Dandelion seeds are equipped
to travel with down parachutes that help them
fly far from the mother plant.

plants with a piece of muslin to prevent the wind from carrying off the seeds. Collect the seeds in the evening, near sunset, when the dampness in the air causes the seed heads to close up. Store the seeds in a cool, dry place in preparation for planting in late fall or early spring.

Sowing Seeds

It takes about 4 pounds of seed to grow 1 acre of the plant spaced about 1 foot apart. This should yield enough seeds for 4 to 5 acres the second year, which will yield 1,000 to 1,500 pounds of dandelion leaves.

Broadcast seeds directly in the ground. From a fall sowing, you will be able to enjoy the greens in spring. Seeds can also be sown directly in the ground in early spring (and they're quite hardy, so no need to wait until after the last frost date). Space the seeds about 12 inches apart and cover them with about ½ inch of soil.

You can also start seeds indoors. Sow the seeds in early spring on the surface of pots or divided plug trays. Cover with a fine layer of perlite. Avoid sowing in seed trays, as the plant's long taproot will make it difficult to remove. Seeds germinate in three to six weeks. For container gardening, pots must be very deep to accommodate the long roots.

Root Division

Dandelions can also be propagated by root division. This method is best done in spring or fall where there is a cluster of dandelions. With a shovel, slice around the perimeter of a plant's root system and lift under the base of the plant, roots and all. By hand, divide the clumps of roots into smaller clumps and replant in another area. Water well.

Growing Tips

Dandelion is great for people who doubt their ability to grow anything, as it is a tenacious plant. Put in some dandelions—they'll boost your green-thumb confidence. Following are a few tips for getting the most out of your crop.

The wild plant is considered more medicinal than cultivated varieties. Cultivated plants have larger leaves and roots, however, and produce more leaves. To make them less bitter, some people like to blanch the leaves by placing a flowerpot upside down over the growing plant. Blanching reduces the nutritional content, however, as a dark green color indicates the presence of chlorophyll and carotenoids. Cultivated leaves tend to be thicker, more tender, and less bitter than those of the wild varieties, as well as lighter in color.

Here are a few other helpful tips:

If you are growing dandelion as **salad greens**, pick off the buds to prevent flowering; this will keep the greens from becoming bitter.

In late fall, dig up dandelion roots, plant them in wooden crates of soil, and store them in a basement or another cool, dark area. If you water them regularly, you'll have **blanched leaves** throughout winter. Remember, though, that while blanching reduces the bitterness, it also decreases nutrient content.

To make a copper-rich garden **fertilizer**, pick three dandelion plants—roots, leaves, stems, and flowers—and place in a bucket with 1 quart of boiling water. Let steep for a half hour. Strain out and compost the spent plant material and use the liquid to water plants.

A trick for growing and harvesting your own **dandelion roots** is to plant the herbs on a narrow bed of loose soil to which some sawdust or wood chips have been added to make the soil more porous. Roots will then be easier to harvest.

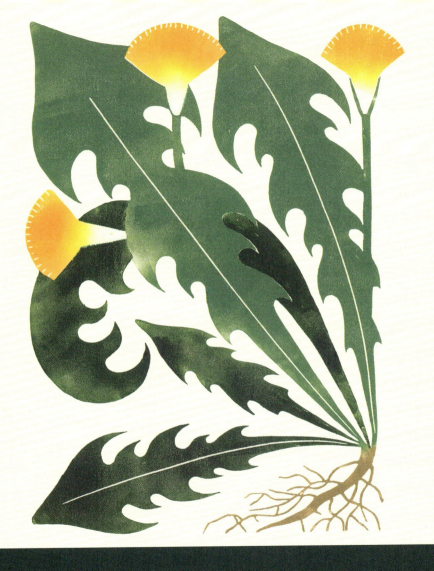

Dandelion is rarely attacked by disease or pests, making it a good candidate for **organic gardening**.

Harvesting Dandelions

Gather dandelions only from environmentally clean areas at least 50 feet away from busy roads and where no pesticides have been used. The roots will be easiest to harvest after a good rain or a few hours after a yard has been watered. If your neighbors don't live on a busy street and don't spray their lawns, ask permission to collect their dandelions—your neighbors will likely be delighted. Then bring them some dandelion muffins to show your gratitude.

Should you live where dandelions simply don't grow, such as in a high-rise apartment building, check your local supermarket, farmers' market, or natural foods store. Nowadays, many retail grocery stores carry dandelions in their produce departments.

Leaves and Stems

Dandelion leaves are best collected in spring before the plants flower. People who claim to dislike the taste of the greens have likely collected the leaves after a plant has flowered, when the greens have turned bitter. Cut the leaves at their base with a knife or snap them off with your fingers. Wash the leaves before using them, as you would with any garden crop. But if you wash the leaves and don't expect to preserve (see page 50) or use them right away, be sure to dry them well to discourage mold. After the plant has seeded, there will be a new growth of leaves later in the summer and these also can be collected. Avoid leaves that are yellow and wilted.

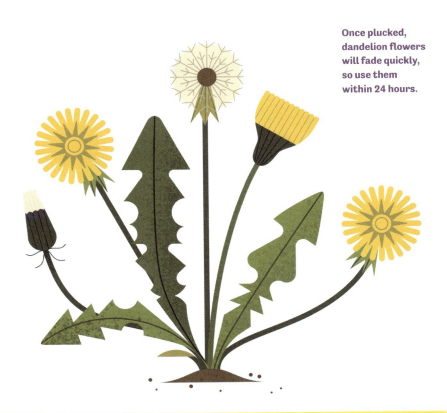

Once plucked, dandelion flowers will fade quickly, so use them within 24 hours.

The dandelion is the greatest natural agent of decoration in our part of America. In some fields it is so abundant that there is no more than enough grass visible to give to it a setting. It is so thoroughly at home that we feel it to be the most prominent and persistent native American, whatever its origin. Coming as it does in the early spring, it clothes an entire landscape with its gorgeous color and rejoices the heart of man . . . it is our tulip in the grass.

—Wallace Nutting, *Connecticut Beautiful,* 1923

The stems are best when the plant is in bloom. Stems are not commonly used as a food, but the sap they contain can be applied to warts to help make them disappear!

Flowers

When collecting flowers, it is handy to have small children with you—they'll love to help. Spread the blossoms on a large cloth so that the insects crawl and fly away before you bring the blooms inside. For appearance and efficacy, I recommend using the flowers the same day they have been collected. Once plucked, dandelion flowers will fade quickly, so use them within 24 hours.

Float flower petals on soup or in punch bowls, or sprinkle on desserts before serving.

Roots

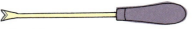

A wonderful hand tool called a dandelion digger (available at gardening supply shops) makes it easier to extract the deep dandelion taproots. To obtain large roots, gather plants that are at least two years old. The best roots will be found in unmowed patches of land and in soil that is rich and loose. Here the root is likely to be single and juicy. (In poorer soil, the root tends to be forked and tough.) The plant is most effective in its fresh state. Roots from older plants will be leathery to eat but can still be used for medicine and in teas.

The ideal times to collect roots are in early spring before the plant flowers and again in fall after the first frost.

Spring harvest. Spring-harvested roots are sweeter than those taken in fall, as they are higher in fructose; less bitter and fibrous; and higher in taraxacin, which stimulates bile

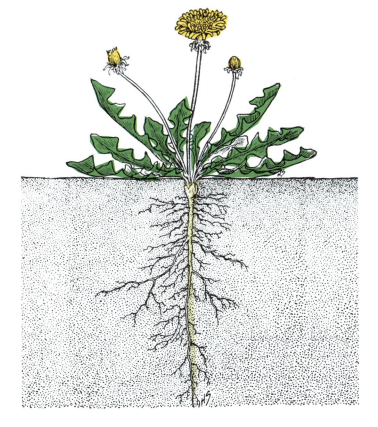

production. But they must be collected before the flower buds are big; otherwise, all their energy will go into producing the blossom, which will deplete the root.

Fall harvest. Roots harvested in fall are more bitter and richer in inulin, which makes them more of a therapeutic medicine. This is partly because during the growing season, the fructose (also known as levulose) in the roots converts to inulin. The winter freeze then breaks down the inulin back to fructose, which sweetens the spring roots.

Gathering Guidelines for Collecting Wild Plants

Learning to grow or collect wild plants—
including dandelions—from your area will greatly
enhance your connection to the earth.
Save time, money, gas, the bees, your health and the planet's!
Here are a few general tips for gathering plants safely
and respectfully.

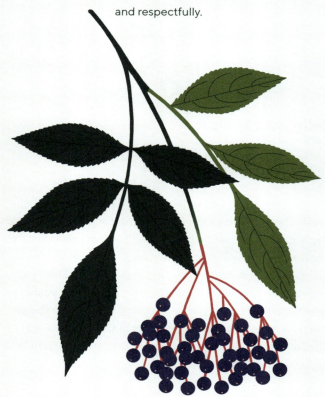

Carefully Identify All Plants

Confirm that you are collecting the proper species, be sure you haven't collected any unwanted plants along with the species you intended to harvest, and identify and leave behind any known endangered species. Use a good guidebook to identify plants. Other places to learn about wild plants are through garden centers, nature centers, and botanical gardens.

If you have a knowledgeable herbalist in your area, you might hire that person to come to your property and flag edible plants with wooden stakes or ice-pop sticks on which you can write each plant's name with permanent ink. That way you can observe your plants for several seasons and really get to know them.

Be Respectful and Joyful

Ask permission from landowners before gathering plants on private land. Ask permission from the herbs you gather, and give thanks. My friend Debra St. Claire likes to remind people, "Bless it before you pick it."

Never take more than 10 percent of what's there. Leave some plants for the wild animals and other aspiring herbalists! Also, it is kinder to take a whole leaf rather than tear a leaf. Collect plants when they are in their prime, not fading. Sing while collecting! Be joyful!

Harvest with the Future in Mind

Collect plants in a way to ensure the continued survival of the species. For example, if all you need are the leaves and flowers, take only some tops. Cutting a plant back can actually help to promote new growth. Leave roots to continue their growing cycle. Also help "thin" plants growing too closely together so that the other plants have more room. Vary the places that you collect from.

Taking a root usually destroys the life cycle of a plant, unlike taking leaves, flowers, or seeds. It is best to collect roots in fall, after the seeds ripen. Then the seeds can be replanted to continue the plant's survival. Cover holes after digging roots, and replant some of the ripe seeds, if the plant has produced them.

Identify the grandfather/mother plant (the tallest, strongest, first to bloom) and leave it in place to ensure the continuation of the strongest of the species.

Harvest at the Best Time

Gather leaves and flowers in morning, after the dew has risen and before the sun is hot. If possible, spray or water plants the day before collecting, to rinse off any residue and give the plants time to dry. Leaves are best taken before the plants begin to flower, as the plants will still be directing energy to the leaves. Flowers are best gathered when just starting to open. Leaves and flowers are usually harvested during the time of the full moon. Roots are said to be best collected during the time of the new moon.

Barks are best collected in spring or fall. If taken after a spell of damp weather, they will separate more easily. Never girdle a tree, as this will impair the sap's ability to rise. Gums and resins are best gathered in hot, dry weather.

Gather Safely

Avoid collecting plants within 50 feet of a busy road or in sprayed or polluted areas. Quality ingredients are essential to creating a high-quality final product. Any final herb preparation should taste and smell like the original plant; herbs that have lost their color and aroma have also lost much of their therapeutic value.

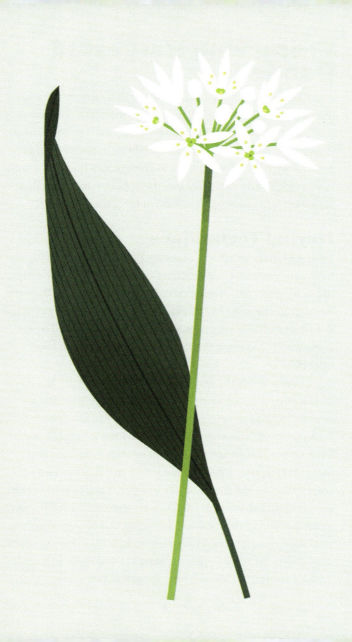

Preserving Harvested Dandelions

Foods that are preserved in such a way that they can remain on a shelf for decades are lacking life force. There are many methods of preserving dandelions so that their nutritional and therapeutic benefits can be enjoyed through the cold winter months until they are available as fresh plants the next spring. Preserving dandelions gives you the opportunity to use this valuable plant year-round as food or medicine.

Drying Techniques

Drying herbs is an age-old technique that safely preserves the herb and creates an end product that is lightweight for carrying or storing. Dehydrating can preserve the flavor of the herb while protecting the enzymes and many of the nutrients of the raw plant and reducing bacterial activity. Dehydrated herbs require only one-sixth the storage space of the fresh plant material.

Leaves. Rinse the leaves and blot dry or collect the day after a rain, after the plant has dried. Place the leaves in a warm, dry, shady, well-ventilated location (an attic or other warm room with good air circulation is ideal). Gather leaves in small bundles secured with a rubber band or string and hang them upside down; lay them on a nylon or stainless steel screen; or put them loosely in a paper bag that has been punched with many holes to allow air circulation. Drying herbs in a paper bag in the back seat of the car can be very effective.

Given the right conditions, leaves will dry in four to seven days. Once crispy-dry, store the leaves in a glass jar in a cool, dark location. They should keep for one to two years.

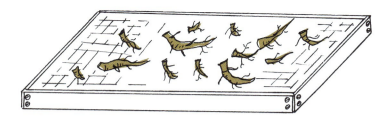

Roots. Drying is the best method of preserving roots. To prepare the roots, scrub them well and slice the largest roots lengthwise so that the insides dry properly. Do not slice the roots before scrubbing, or the valuable milky juice will be washed away.

Once washed, place the roots on a screen and set in a warm, dry, shady, well-ventilated area. They should dry within 3 to 14 days, depending on the size of the roots and the humidity of the air. Alternatively, you can dry them in a dehydrator set to 120°F (50°C). You can also dry roots in the oven, if you have one that can be set to a low enough temperature. Preheat the oven to 120°F (50°C) and set the roots directly on the racks. Keep the oven door slightly ajar. Once dried (in 4 to 12 hours, depending on the size), store the roots in a glass jar in a cool, dry place. They will keep for about a year.

Storing

Clean, dry glass jars are the best ways to store dried herbs for maximum shelf life. Place the herbs in labeled and dated airtight jars soon after they are dried, so they don't collect dust and cobwebs, and store them away from heat and light. Heat, air, moisture, and light will cause herbs to degrade more rapidly. Because of that, I use dark amber bottles whenever possible.

Freezing

Collect dandelion leaves and wash them well. Steam them for 1½ minutes in a covered colander over a saucepan containing a few inches of boiling water. Then stop the cooking by plunging the greens into cold water. Drain well, then pack into containers and freeze.

Alternatively, put the fresh greens into ziplock bags, squeeze out the excess air, seal, and freeze or freeze in densely packed plastic containers. Frozen greens are suitable for use in recipes that call for cooked greens.

Canning

Wash dandelions (greens or roots), chop, and steam in a bit of water until wilted. Pack into clean canning jars, leaving ½ inch of headroom. Add ½ teaspoon salt to each pint jar or 1 teaspoon salt to each quart. Cover with boiling water, leaving ½ inch of headroom. Screw on the lids. Process in a pressure cooker at 10 pounds of pressure for 70 minutes for pints, 90 minutes for quarts. Make sure the lids' seals are tight when the jars have cooled. For those that do not seal properly, refrigerate and use them within three days.

Sales of fresh **dandelion greens** in the United States are estimated to be in the millions of dollars, with New Jersey, Arizona, California, Florida, and Texas known for growing dandelions on a commercial scale. In fact, Vineland, New Jersey, considers itself the Dandelion Capital of the World.

Dandelion Vinegar

Use dandelion vinegar in marinades and dressings, mix it in a bit of hot water (with honey if you desire) and sip to chase away a cold or flu, or stir it into herbal mustards. Dandelion vinegar can also be added to the bath to soothe itchy or sunburned skin or applied as a hair rinse for body and shine.

Be sure to use sterilized jars and lids for your vinegars. (Washing the jars and lids in the dishwasher with high heat should do the trick.) Vinegar can be corrosive, so if you use metal lids instead of plastic ones, place a layer of wax paper (cut a bit larger than the jar lid) between the lid and the jar to prevent rust from developing.

To make a vinegar, fill a clean glass jar two-thirds full of washed, chopped dandelion leaves. Cover to the top with raw apple cider vinegar, making sure all the leaves are submerged in the vinegar, and stir. Screw on the jar's plastic lid or slip a piece of wax paper under a metal lid. Allow it to steep for one month, then strain through a paint strainer bag (available at paint or hardware stores). Avoid squeezing the bag, or too much sediment will leak through, making the vinegar look cloudy. Pour into pretty bottles and label. Vinegar will keep for one year.

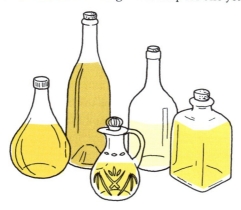

Too Many Dandelions?

The first crop of dandelions is a cheerful sign of spring. But perhaps you have a few too many and you'd like to welcome other plants as well. Clipping the dandelion blossoms will discourage seeds from forming and thus decrease the plant's ability to spread. Use the harvested dandelion blossoms for food and medicine, of course. Better yet—dig up the excess plants and use the roots for tea and food and make wine from the flowers! Using a dandelion digger or trowel, uproot the plant in spring when it's in flower but before seeds begin to form. At this point, the energy of the plant is aboveground and the food reserve in the root is less strong. If you leave a small piece of root in the ground, another dandelion will still come up. However, repeated diggings will eventually deplete the plant's food supply and cause it to lose its grip on life.

A Final Plea for the Dandelion

Perhaps your neighborhood association, unenlightened, is pressuring you to get rid of the dandelions in your yard. Share with a few neighbors some recipes and a copy of this book, and start your own dandelion revolution! If this doesn't warm some hearts, remind people of the damage that herbicides cause to our planet. Spray programs are dangerous to animals and humans as well as to plants, and they poison our precious water supplies. Instead of chemicals, put some glitter in your yard—the golden flowers of the delightful dandelion.

Isn't it time we learned to love and utilize the friendly dandelion? It offers itself freely, with something for everyone. Welcome this beautiful and useful plant. The people who tend to be the most aggressive about dandelions—angry, wanting to

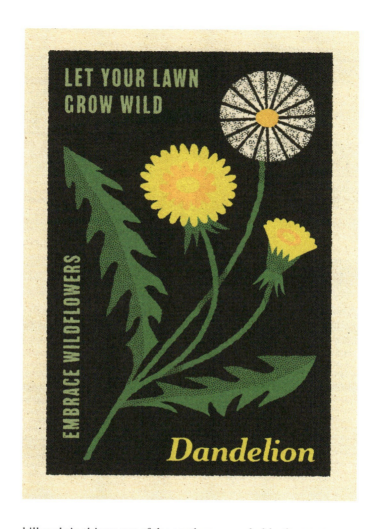

LET YOUR LAWN
GROW WILD

EMBRACE WILDFLOWERS

Dandelion

kill and rip things out of the earth—are probably the ones who could most benefit from this plant. Since you can't beat 'em, eat 'em—and enjoy the numerous health benefits.

Celebrate life and enjoy dandelions!

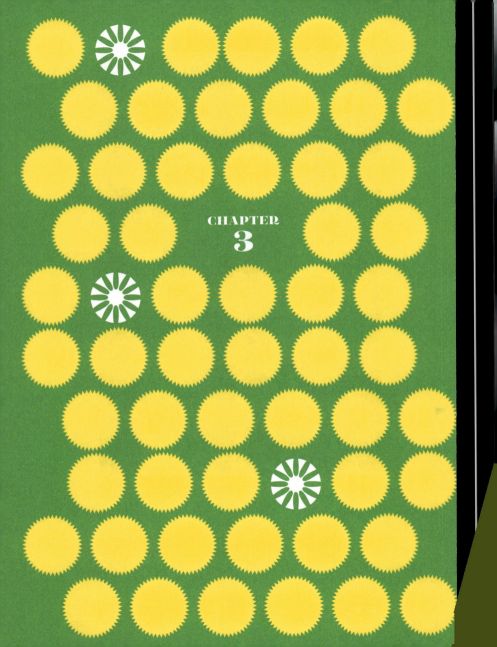

CHAPTER
3

Traditional Uses of DANDELION MEDICINE

Dandelions have served humanity for thousands of years. The Greek naturalist Theophrastus (c. 372–287 BCE) marveled at the dandelion's ability to flower over and over and recommended that the herb be taken as a tonic. In the Jewish tradition, dandelion leaves were one of the five bitter herbs of Passover mentioned in the Bible (Exodus). When Roman legions invaded Gaul and the Rhineland, they were delighted to find dandelions growing there. The Celts claimed dandelion as their own, relishing it to make food and wine. The Anglo-Saxon tribes that settled in the British Isles after the withdrawal of the Romans used dandelion to prevent scurvy and as a diuretic and laxative.

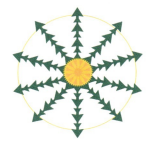

Early Western Traditions

The Islamic physician Ibn Sina, known in the West as Avicenna (980–1037 CE), prescribed dandelion root to stimulate bile production for those with liver problems. Herbalists in thirteenth-century Myddfai, a village in Wales, wrote about the health benefits of dandelion. In a 1485 European herbal, the *Ortus Sanitatis*, dandelion is mentioned as a medicinal plant. Nicholas Culpeper, an English herbalist of the seventeenth century, suggested dandelion for "every evil disposition of the body," which led to dandelion being considered "the official remedy for disorders." Culpeper also wrote of the dandelion: "You see here what virtues this common herb hath, and it is the reason the French and Dutch so often eat them in the spring; and now if you look a little farther, you may plainly see without a pair of spectacles, that foreign physicians are not so selfish as ours are, but communicative of the virtues of plants to people."

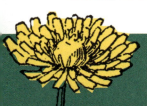

Heartburn Remedy

Here's a common remedy from the Ojibwe tradition for treating heartburn: Boil a handful of flowers until the water turns yellow, let it steep overnight, strain out the flowers, and give the liquid first thing in the morning; continue treatment for one month.

NORTH AMERICAN USES

Though the dandelion is not native to North America, it is believed that the plants may have arrived with the Vikings as early as 100 CE. Over time, it became part of the food and medicine traditions of the Indigenous nations of North America.

Members of the Apache nation collect it for days before their spring feasts.

✳

Indigenous groups in the Great Basin region and the Tohono O'odham of the Southwest eat dandelions both raw and cooked.

✳

The Iroquois boil the leaves with fatty meats.

✳

Many Indigenous North American nations also use dandelion medicinally.

✳

Mohegans drink a tea of dandelion leaf as a liver tonic.

✳

Kiowa women boil dandelion flowers with pennyroyal leaves to treat menstrual cramps.

✳

Women of the Tohono O'odham nation also use a tea of the flowers for menstrual cramps.

✳

In the Navajo tradition, a tea of the root is made for a new mother following birthing, to hasten the delivery of the placenta.

✳

Mohegans and Potawatomi people prepare the root as a tonic tea.

Members of the Nuxalk Nation of Bella Coola, British Columbia, and of the Ojibwe nation use dandelion root as a remedy for both stomachache and heartburn.

✳

In the medicinal tradition of the Delaware nation, a dandelion root tea is given as a laxative and tonic.

✳

Iroquois people use dandelion to treat jaundice.

✳

Meskwaki healers use a tea of the root to treat chest pains, and Tewa healers use a poultice of the leaves to help heal broken bones, bruises, swellings, sores, and fractures.

✳

In the medicinal practices of many Indigenous nations, the juice from the stem is applied to bee stings. The flowers are also used to make a yellow dye for deerskin.

✳

Many groups traditionally chewed various plants as a gum to moisten their mouths. Dandelion stems, because of their latex content, were used in this way. The young plant was regarded by many as having mild narcotic properties, too.

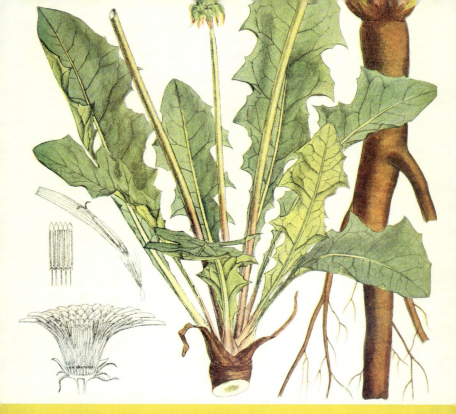

Love Charm

Historically, an Iroquois woman would select a dandelion with a particularly long taproot that had a fork and a small appendage resembling a part of the male anatomy. Then the name of her intended beloved was spoken several times and the root thrown behind her to ensure that her love soon would follow. Also as a love charm, dandelion roots that were found growing entwined would be boiled in water. When the water cooled, it was splashed on the face to make the user sexually irresistible.

Early European Colonists

Dandelion continued to spread across North America, carried by early European colonists who settled along the Atlantic coast. They brought dandelion seeds to grow in their gardens, to remind them of home, and fenced the precious plants to keep out gophers. As forests were cut down, dandelion seeds escaped to grow where room was now abundant.

In the 1800s, Europeans arriving in the Midwest planted dandelion to provide food for bees, and dandelion's spread across the continent continued. By the time of the Civil War, people across the country used the plant as food and medicine, especially when regular food supplies were cut off by blockades. They also substituted the roasted roots for coffee, a practice that continued after the war.

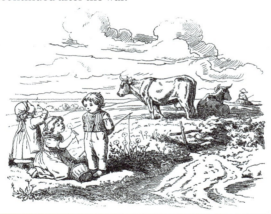

Yellow japanned buttercups and star-disked dandelions, just as we see them lying in the grass, like sparks that have leaped from the kindling sun of summer; . . .

—Oliver Wendell Holmes, *The Professor at the Breakfast Table*

Twentieth-Century Traditions

Dandelion was an official herb in the early pharmacopoeia of the United States. The root was considered the significant part of the plant from 1831 to 1926 and was included in the National Formulary until 1965.

Dandelion is still included in the pharmacopoeias of Hungary, Poland, Russia, and Switzerland. Russians referred to dandelions as "the elixir of life," and it was a favorite remedy of the imperial court from the time of Peter the Great until the early 1900s. In rural Russia, dandelion root is still used to treat tuberculosis and prevent miscarriage.

During World Wars I and II, health departments in both the United States and Europe publicized this herb as a healthful food. Before World War I, dandelions were cultivated in Germany, and the exported roots were as large as parsnips. By World War II, England had stopped growing many herbs, feeling it was cheaper to import them, yet when their supplies were cut off, the British Ministry of Health organized teams of women to collect dandelions. Honored for its war service, the dandelion was given a place in the British Pharmacopoeia.

During World War II, when many people throughout Europe suffered nutritional deficiencies, Italian housewives in small villages would brew up a pot of dandelion soup and leave it on a windowsill as nourishment for impoverished passersby. Dandelion flowers were also chopped and added to margarine to give it the appearance of butter.

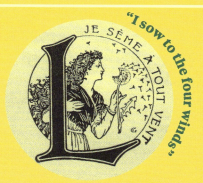

Throughout the twentieth century and in popular culture today, a wide range of cultures have devised many uses for dandelion for a range of purposes:

Lydia Pinkham, a renowned Quaker nurse, herbalist, and business-woman of the mid-nineteenth and early twentieth centuries, included dandelion root in the original recipe for her famous **women's tonic**.

The Eclectic physicians of the early 1900s, who combined herbal and modern medicine, regarded dandelion as beneficial for **autointoxication** (clearing toxins out of the body).

A popular Dutch legend says that if you eat **dandelion salad** on Mondays and Thursdays, you will be healthy always.

In Japan, dandelions are cultivated as an **ornamental plant**. Japanese breeders have produced two hundred colorful varieties in white, orange, copper, and black.

Dandelions have long been a favorite **spring vegetable** of Mennonites and the Amish.

In Germany, there is a custom of eating a bowl of **dandelion greens** on the day before Good Friday (called by some "green Thursday"), in the belief that eating them on that day will ensure good health for the rest of the year.

There is a French expression that translates to "eating dandelion by the roots," which means the same as the American expression "pushing up daisies"; it implies that someone is dead.

Dandelion in Chinese Medicine

Dandelion grows abundantly in China, especially in the Yangtze River valley, and records from the Tang dynasty date its use back to at least the seventh century. In China, a related species, *Taraxacum mongolicum*, which is called pú gong ying, is used to "clear heat" or treat infections or "fire poisons" as well as to clear dampness. The Chinese also call their dandelion huang-hua ti-ting, meaning "yellow-flowered herb," or chian-nou-ts'ao, meaning "plowing and hoeing weed."

The Liver System

In traditional Chinese medicine, dandelion is often used to treat the liver, which governs circulation of blood and is important in maintaining a smooth flow of chi, or life energy, through the body. Dandelion tea made from the entire plant is used for any "hot" disorder that manifests in excess "heat" in the liver.

According to traditional Chinese medicine, the liver system is associated with anger and depression. As you begin to use dandelion, stored emotions that you thought you had forgotten may arise and become stirred up before leaving your body. On the other hand, dandelion root can be prescribed to clear stored, negative emotions.

THE HERB OF MANY USES

Dandelion is officially recognized in the pharmacopoeia of China, and practitioners of traditional Chinese medicine have used dandelion to treat an incredible assortment of ailments and illnesses, including the following.

- Abscesses, boils, carbuncles, and sores
- Appendicitis
- Breast cancer, lack of milk production, mastitis, and tumors
- Chronic pelvic inflammatory disease
- Colds, fevers, and pneumonia
- Coughs and bronchitis
- Dental problems
- Eye inflammation
- Food poisoning
- Hemorrhoids
- Hepatitis
- Inflammation of the gums, mouth, and throat
- Insect bites
- Itchy skin
- Jaundice
- Mumps
- Pancreatitis
- Snakebites
- Tonsillitis
- Ulcers

Ayurvedic Medicine

Ayurveda, translated as "life science," is the traditional system of healing in India that has become popular worldwide. It's based on mind-body-spirit connections that address specific body and energy types. In Ayurveda, dandelion is considered an herb that helps purge ama (accumulated waste and toxins) from the body. It nurtures the air element (vata) and decreases fire (pitta) and water (kapha), and thus should be used with caution by those with extreme vata constitutions. As in traditional Chinese medicine, dandelion is thought of as bitter, sweet, and cooling.

Specific Uses

In Ayurvedic practice, dandelion is taken to address stagnation of energy in the liver and gallbladder and helps cleanse bile ailments as well as breast problems such as tumors, insufficient milk production, cysts, and swollen lymph glands. Dandelion leaf is used most often for acute conditions and the root for chronic conditions, such as boils, carbuncles, gout, and cancer.

Ayurvedic medicine holds that dandelion is safe and beneficial for appetite loss and poor digestion, as it improves assimilation. It is also used for gynecological problems such as pelvic inflammatory disease and endometriosis. It is considered astringent, strengthening to the entire body, a cooling energy tonic, and beneficial in treating infection.

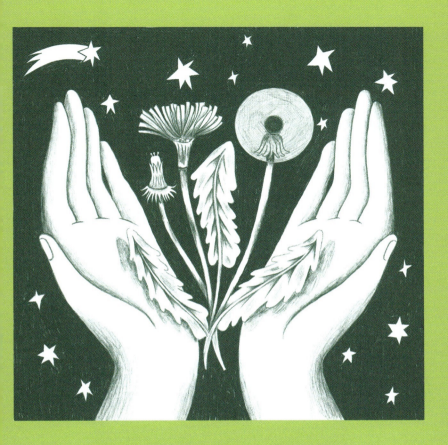

Until the twentieth century, there existed a
National Dandelion Society.
Maybe it's time for a comeback!
In the past decade, people in England have
expressed concern over the possibility of the dandelion
becoming extinct because of herbicide use.

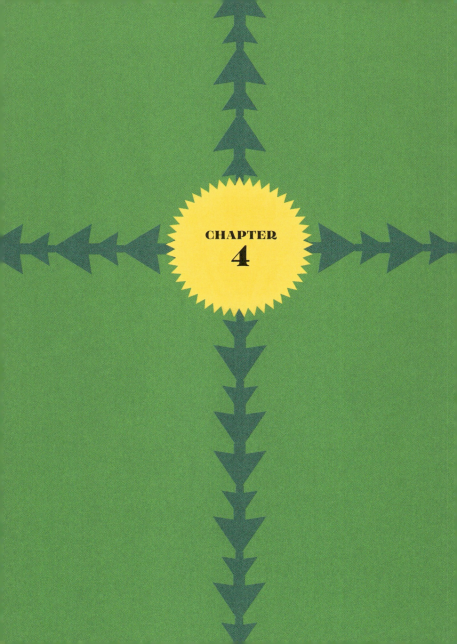

CHAPTER
4

Dandelion's
MEDICINAL PROPERTIES

As a medicinal plant, dandelion is a self-contained pharmacy. It is one of the most widely used herbal medicines in the world. The systems primarily affected by dandelion are the liver, kidneys, gallbladder, pancreas, intestines, and blood. It is held in particularly high regard as one of the safest and most important herbs for the liver.

A Cure-All for What Ails You

Dandelion has been used to cure just about everything, at any given time and place, and can be taken in a number of different ways. Dandelion root is most medicinal in the unroasted form and may be taken in a tea, in an extract, or in capsule form. Leaves are also commonly offered as medicine and may be used fresh or dried in the form of tea, tincture, and capsules. Fresh stems provide sap, which has medicinal properties, too. The flowers are best used fresh and serve mainly as a food source.

The leaves, with their mineral-rich properties, can nourish bones (warding off osteoporosis) and teeth. Drinking dandelion leaf tea over time helps increase joint mobility and reduce stiffness, decrease serum cholesterol and uric acid, and promote digestive regularity. Drinking a tea of the roots after giving birth aids in the expulsion of the placenta. In Germany, dandelion juice from the stem and root is taken internally to improve eye health; the plant is sometimes referred to as eye root. In China, dandelion leaf is used internally to treat styes and conjunctivitis. Dandelions have long been used in cancer treatment; they are rich in chlorophyll and antioxidants like beta-carotene and flavonoids.

Dandelions for Better Sight?

In the human body, the beta-carotene from dandelion greens is converted to 11-cis-retinol, a metabolite of vitamin A and the most important constituent of rhodopsin, a protein in the retina's rods (the cells that enable us to see in low-light conditions).

Giving Life to the Liver

Dandelion is a time-tested detoxifier and strengthener of the liver. Because the liver is the organ responsible for breaking down and clearing excess hormones from the body, one of the reasons that dandelion can improve menstrual problems is related to enhanced liver function.

Dandelion root is rich in phytosterols, so it is also excellent to use during menopause to alleviate hot flashes. It helps the liver break down excess luteinizing hormones and follicle-stimulating hormones. A menopausal woman on hormone replacement therapy can take dandelion to nourish, protect, and support the liver while taking the pharmaceuticals.

According to the principles of natural medicine in many cultures, the emotional body is affected by the physical body. The liver is said to correspond to the emotions of anger, depression, and creativity. Like other herbs that influence the liver, dandelion helps relieve anger, depression, jealousy, oversensitivity, and resentment. So think of this plant as both physically and emotionally beneficial: so much healing power with no harmful side effects!

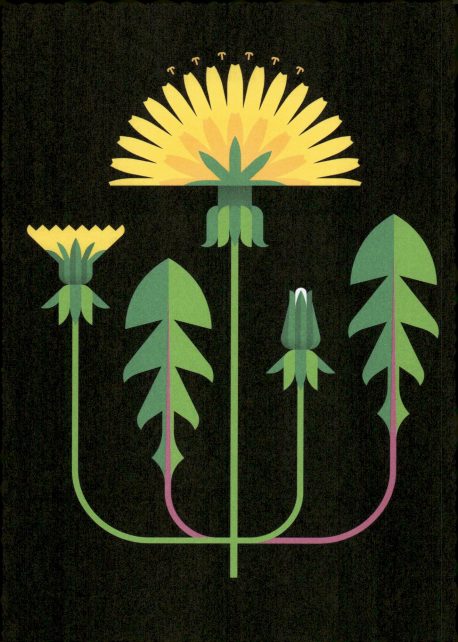

Clinical Trials and Scientific Findings

Clinical studies to introduce a new drug can cost millions of dollars and are affordable only to large pharmaceutical companies, which hope to regain their expenditure when the new drug is released for sale. Understandably, then, there haven't been many studies on the medicinal value of an herb that grows so wild and free and is almost always readily available. However, dandelion has been used by millions of people for thousands of years. And over the past hundred years, the studies that have been conducted have served to confirm dandelion's beneficial properties.

Dandelion's positive effects on the liver are due primarily to its ability to increase bile production by causing the gallbladder to contract, releasing stored bile and its high choline content, which acts as a tonic for the liver. As author and herbalist Christopher Hobbs reports, in a 1938 Italian study 12 subjects suffering liver dysfunction symptoms such as jaundice and low energy were injected with 5 milliliters of dandelion extract daily for 20 days. Cholesterol and urinary bilirubin were measured before and after administering the dandelion. Although the standards for testing are much more vigorous in modern times, 11 of the 12 subjects enjoyed a significant lowering of cholesterol levels and all 12 reported feeling better.

According to K. Faber, author of "The Dandelion *Taraxacum officinale*," clinical trials in China from the mid-1900s proved dandelion to be effective against bronchitis, pneumonia, tonsillitis, and other respiratory disorders.

In a 1950 study conducted by L. Kroeber in England, dandelion was a successful remedy for hepatitis, jaundice, and liver enlargement, all common symptoms of liver dysfunction.

Dandelion has a long tradition of being a weight-loss herb for humans, which prompted researchers to study these claims on animals. In a 1974 Romanian study conducted by Erzsébet Rácz-Kotilla, Gábor Rácz, and A. Solomon, rats and mice were given 50 milliliters of a dandelion infusion per every kilogram of body weight for one month. During this period, they lost as much as 30 percent of their original weight. The loss was due to the diuretic activity of dandelion, the mild laxative effect, and the enhancing of liver function. The study's authors postulated that part of dandelion's weight loss–enhancing effect comes from its gland-stimulating qualities.

According to a 1979 study from Japan by K. K. Kotobuki Seiyaku, when the polysaccharide and aqueous extracts of dandelion have been administered to animals, they exhibit antitumor activity.

In the book *Chinese Herbal Medicine: Materia Medica*, Dan Bensky, Andrew Gamble, and Ted Kaptchuk detail studies conducted in China indicating that dandelion has in vitro antibacterial effects against *Staphylococcus aureus*, *Streptococcus pneumoniae*, *Pseudomonas aeruginosa*, *Shigella* species, *Corynebacterium diphtheriae*, and *Neisseria meningitidis*.

Dandelion's constituent inulin has shown positive hypoglycemic activity—meaning it helps stabilize blood sugar levels—in animals. Inulin is composed of chains of fructose, which may possibly act to buffer the blood's levels of glucose and prevent sudden fluctuations.

A 2014 study in China showed that dandelion had a protective effect on liver cells and an antiviral effect against the hepatitis B virus. Science is validating what the ancient ones have known for centuries.

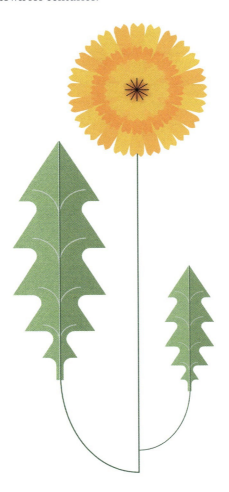

Medicinal Properties of Dandelion

PART	PROPERTY	ACTION/EVIDENCE
Root, leaf	Alterative	Helps purify the blood by increasing blood flow to the tissues, aiding assimilation and stimulating metabolism.
Root	Antibilious	Helps remove excess bile from the system.
Root	Anti-inflammatory	Reduces inflammation, such as glandular swelling.
Root	Antibacterial	Inhibits the growth of germs.
Root, sap	Antifungal	Inhibits fungal growth.
Root	Cholagogue	Causes the gallbladder to contract and release stored bile from the liver. Can be used in cases of congestion of the liver and gallbladder.
Root	Choleretic	Stimulates bile production and increases cleansing of the bile duct.
Root	Deobstruent	Moves obstructions, especially those originating in the liver.
Root, sap	Discutient	Helps dissolve abnormal growths.
Root, flower	Hepatic	Strengthens and tonifies the liver.
Root	Hypnotic	Induces a deep, healing sleep state.
Root	Laxative	Improves bowel movements.
Root	Lipotropic	Prevents the accumulation of fat in the liver by stimulating bile production.
Root, leaf	Lithotriptic	Helps dissolve and discharge urinary and gallbladder stones.
Root	Purgative	Increases bile secretions that activate intestinal peristalsis.
Root, leaf	Restorative	Helps in the renewal and repair of organs and can help prevent further destruction. Also restorative to connective tissue.
Root	Sedative	Quiets the nerves.

It would be difficult to think of a plant exhibiting more medicinal properties than does the dandelion. Here are some of its amazing effects.

PART	PROPERTY	ACTION/EVIDENCE
Leaf, sap, flower	Anodyne	Lessens nerve excitability, thus relieving pain.
Leaf	Antacid	Relieves stomach acid.
Leaf	Antilithic	Helps prevent and discharge urinary and biliary stones and gravel.
Leaf	Antioxidant	Helps the body resist free-radical damage thanks to high levels of beta-carotene and vitamin C.
Leaf, root	Antirheumatic	Root helps disperse acidic deposits in the joints; leaves help gout and rheumatism as well as glandular swellings.
Leaf, root	Antitumor	Although there is little clinical data, dandelion has traditionally been used as a poultice to reduce tumors; in traditional Chinese medicine, dandelion poultices are used to treat breast cancer.
Leaf, root	Aperient	Works as a mild laxative.
Leaf, root	Astringent	Tightens and tones tissue. Helps dry excessive secretions.
Leaf, root	Bitter	Stimulates the initial stages of digestion, including increasing saliva production and gastric juice activity as well as bile release.
Leaf	Decongestant	Helps open respiratory passages and improve breathing.
Leaf, root	Depurative	Helps cleanse and purify the body.
Leaf, root	Digestive	Increases hydrochloric acid levels in the stomach. All the glands in the digestive system respond quickly to dandelion.
Leaf, root	Diuretic	Stimulates the flow of urine, so helps reduce fluid retention. Helpful in cases of fluid retention due to heart problems.
Leaf	Febrifuge	Helps lower fever.

PART	PROPERTY	ACTION/EVIDENCE
Leaf, root	Galactagogue	Increases mother's milk.
Leaf, root	Immune stimulant	Can be used for acute infections such as tonsillitis and pelvic inflammatory disease.
Leaf	Laxative	Increases bowel function.
Leaf	Narcotic (mild)	Helps relieve pain and induce sleep.
Leaf	Nutritive	Supplies lots of nutrients; builds and tones the body.
Leaf, root	Stomachic	Strengthens and tonifies the stomach. Improves digestion and relieves gas.
Leaf, root	Tonic	Promotes general health and well-being.
Leaf, flower	Vulnerary	Encourages wound healing by promoting cellular growth and repair.
Flower	Calmative	Is mildly tranquilizing.
Flower	Cardiotonic	Benefits the heart.
Flower	Emollient	Used externally to soothe, soften, and protect the skin.

Avoid using dandelions from lawns that have been sprayed with herbicides or chemical fertilizers in the past two or even three years. The chemicals used to poison this magnificent plant are far more dangerous than this herb ever could be!

Contraindications and Cautions

For most people, dandelion is considered safe even in large amounts; however, as with anything else, there is always the possibility that you could be allergic to it. There are no reports of toxic effects from its internal or external use. Even pregnant women use dandelion leaves, to prevent edema and hypertension. Very few cases have been reported of abdominal discomfort, loose stools, nausea, and heartburn associated with dandelion consumption.

Kommission E, a German panel of experts on drugs and medical devices, allows dandelion leaf and root for their diuretic effects, as a cholagogue and appetite stimulant, and for dyspepsia, and they are an approved over-the-counter drug. Kommission E feels dandelion to be contraindicated for obstruction of the bile duct, and suggests that it be used for gallstones only after consulting with a physician. In the United States, dandelion is considered GRAS (Generally Regarded as Safe); in the United Kingdom, dandelion is on the General Sales List; in Canada, it is approved as an over-the-counter drug; and in France, it is classified as a traditional medicine.

The fresh latex in the stems can cause contact dermatitis in some sensitive individuals. Consult with a physician prior to using dandelion if you suffer from an obstructed bile duct or gallstones. Some individuals with gastric hyperacidity may find excessive use of dandelion leaf aggravating. To modify some of the cooling and contracting effects of dandelion when it is used over a long period, mix it with a small amount of ginger and licorice root.

Benefits for Specific Ailments and Conditions

Dandelion is often regarded as a blood purifier, which aids in the process of filtering and straining wastes from the blood-stream. It is useful in treating obstructions of the gallbladder, liver, pancreas, and spleen. The vulnerary, tonic, astringent, and antimicrobial properties of dandelion also make it helpful in the treatment of prostate problems. The leaves aid in the elimination of uric acid. Use the root primarily for problems related to the liver, spleen, stomach, and kidneys and the leaf for liver, kidney, and bladder concerns. Dandelion helps address hypertension by decreasing excessive fluids in the body that the heart must pump.

During Pregnancy

When dandelion leaves are ingested during pregnancy, they strengthen the liver and can help prevent preeclampsia, which manifests as high blood pressure with edema. Dandelion helps the fetus develop a strong liver of its own. Being high in iron, the leaves can help prevent anemia, a common concern for pregnant mothers. High blood pressure and fluid retention during pregnancy can both be safely treated with dandelion leaf tea (and improvement in diet).

For Children

Taking dandelion root in the last few weeks of pregnancy will help prevent pathological jaundice in the baby. Should the baby have jaundice, the root—taken as a tea—ideally can be drunk by the nursing mother, or given to the infant directly as the next-best choice. About 1 teaspoon of the tea daily is appropriate for a baby, but the mother can drink as much as she is able. As dandelion leaf is a galactagogue, it increases the nursing mother's milk supply and bolsters its nutritional quality—another boon for the infant! The leaves and root of dandelion make an excellent food or tea rich in minerals for growing children. Because dandelion leaves and roots help cleanse the liver, kidneys, and therefore the blood, they are excellent for teenagers concerned about acne.

Sometimes, when playing with the flowers, children may also eat them. This is fine, in small quantities. If they eat too many, children can become nauseous. Occasionally a child assimilates the diuretic properties through the skin from overhandling the fresh plant and thus may need to urinate more. If this happens, simply give the child a tea of peppermint, fennel seed, and chamomile, and they will begin to feel better.

For recreation, one favorite childhood pastime is making chains of dandelions as necklaces, bracelets, and crowns. Children also often strip the stems of flowers and leaves, split the stems at top and bottom, then drop them in water to watch them curl and twist into pretty shapes.

CHAPTER
5

Making and Using
DANDELION MEDICINES

Dandelion medicine has many benefits. It's safe, effective, abundant, fresh, and free. It's pleasant to use and has a safety record that spans thousands of years of use. Medicinally, dandelions can be used fresh or prepared as a tea, tincture, encapsulated powder, juice, or homeopathic formula. Most dandelion remedies are easy to make at home, and in most regions, the fresh flowers are easy to collect—even, in fact, difficult to avoid tripping over. However, if you have neither the time nor the inclination, you can usually purchase harvested plants, dried leaves and roots, or remedies from natural foods stores, herb shops, or mail-order sources.

Tea Preparations

One of the greatest pleasures is a peaceful, reflective moment spent with a cup of tea. Taking the time to sit quietly over a cup of herbal tea, alone or with loved ones, is psychologically de-stressing, relaxing, and life affirming; in addition, herbal tea is itself extremely healthful and can be healing as well. Think "I'm nourishing myself with the strength of this herb" as you savor any of the recipes that begin on page 87. For medicinal purposes, drink three or four cups daily.

Making Infusions

You can choose from two methods to make a tea from the leaves of plants. The glass-jar method takes longer but produces a stronger tea. The French-press method is quicker, but the resulting infusion is not as strong. In both cases, use ½ ounce of dried leaves or 1 ounce of fresh leaves per cup of water. After steeping, strain and compost the spent leaves.

Glass-jar method. Place the tea ingredients in a glass canning jar. Cover with freshly boiled water. Put on the lid and let steep overnight, then strain out the solids. The glass-jar method takes time but makes a potent tea.

French-press method. Simply place the herbs in a French press and cover with 1 quart of boiling water. Let steep for at least 20 minutes. (If you don't own a French press, first steep the herbs, then strain the tea through a fine-mesh strainer.)

Making Decoctions

A decoction is similar to an infusion but is used to extract constituents from tougher, more fibrous parts of plants, such as roots, tubers, barks, and woody stems. A decoction is necessary to extract the healing properties from the roots of dandelion. Put 1 ounce of chopped dried roots or 2 ounces of chopped fresh roots in a pan with 2 cups of water. Bring to a boil, cover, and simmer for 20 minutes. Strain out and compost the spent roots.

Making Herbal Tinctures

Tinctures are small and portable, making them easy to use when you are at work or school or while traveling. For medicinal purposes, use 30 drops in a bit of hot water three times daily.

Both dandelion leaves and roots can be made into a tincture using 1 part dandelion (by weight) for every 5 parts (by volume) of a 40 percent alcohol solution, such as vodka or brandy. It makes sense to prepare enough tincture to last at least a month, using an ounce as one "part." In addition, any of the tea formulas that follow can easily be made into a tincture. Prepare the herbs by chopping or by grinding in a blender. Pour the

The Dandelion "Cure"

In Europe, many people commonly follow "the cure," which entails drinking three cups of dandelion root tea daily for six to eight weeks. They may do this twice a year, spring and autumn. Another spring cure is to take 1 or 2 tablespoons of dandelion leaf juice in some water at morning and night for several weeks. Consuming dandelion in spring helps counter the ill effects of a winter of eating only cooked, heavy foods. Drink dandelion leaf and root tea when on a cleansing diet or fasting.

formula into a jar large enough to hold your herbs with some extra room. Cover with vodka or brandy, adding an extra inch of the liquor so that the herbs are saturated and completely covered. This will help preserve the herbs and extract both the water-soluble and the alcohol-soluble properties. Shake daily. Strain after a month, first with a fine-mesh strainer and then through a clean undyed cloth, squeezing tightly. Pressing the herbs, while still in the cloth, with a potato ricer can be helpful. Compost the spent herbs and bottle the tincture in dark glass containers. Label and date. Store away from heat and light. Tinctures will keep for two to three years.

Be sure to label and date your tinctures—once arrayed side by side on a pantry shelf, they all begin to look alike.

Dandelion Dosages

Small doses are considered more restorative; large ones are more effective for clearing "heat," such as fever, infection, or inflammation. When using dandelion in the form of medicine, dosage guidelines include:

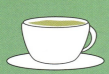

1 cup of tea
three or four
times daily

30 drops of tincture
in a bit of water
three times daily

2 size "00" capsules
three times daily

MEDICINAL TEA RECIPES

The tea recipes on the following pages can be used to treat, soothe, heal, or ease the symptoms of a variety of ailments and conditions. Ingredients are called for in parts, which will enable you to make as much of the recipe as is appropriate for your needs. Note that in the ingredients lists, the term *herb* refers to the aboveground portion of the plant, including the stem, leaf, and flower. And don't forget that the recipes can also be formulated as tinctures for potent yet portable remedies—see Making Herbal Tinctures, page 85.

I usually suggest 1 heaping teaspoon of herb per cup of water. So, for example, if there are four herbs in the formula, you might use 1 teaspoon of each and 1 quart of water.

When making a tea from both leaves and roots, first prepare the roots as a decoction, as instructed on page 84. After 20 minutes of simmering, remove the pan from the heat, add the leaves, cover, and let the mixture steep for at least 10 minutes. Strain out and compost the spent herbs.

Overcoming-Addiction Tea

This tea will lend strength and willpower when you've decided to give up caffeine, nicotine, alcohol, or even something stronger. It strengthens the adrenal glands and cleanses and supports the nerves.

INFUSE

1 part skullcap (*Scutellaria lateriflora*) herb
1 part oat straw (*Avena sativa*) herb

DECOCT

1 part dandelion root
1 part Asian ginseng (*Panax ginseng*) root, chopped or sliced

Allergy-Relief Tea

This formula soothes inflammation and helps the body be more resistant to allergens.

INFUSE

1 part nettle (*Urtica dioica*) leaf
1 part mullein (*Verbascum thapsus*) leaf

DECOCT

1 part dandelion root
1 part marsh mallow (*Althaea officinalis*) root
½ part licorice (*Glycyrrhiza glabra*) root

Improve-Anemia Tea

For those suffering from anemia, this tea is rich in minerals, especially iron, and helps build the blood.

INFUSE

1 part dandelion leaf
1 part nettle (*Urtica dioica*) leaf
1 part watercress (*Nasturtium officinale*) leaf

DECOCT

1 part yellow dock (*Rumex crispus*) root

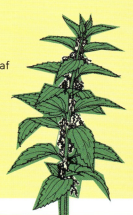

Arthritis-Relief Tea

Ease your joints with this anti-inflammatory preparation. It also helps strengthen the immune system.

INFUSE

1 part nettle (*Urtica dioica*) leaf

DECOCT

1 part dandelion root
1 part yucca (*Yucca glauca*) root
1 part devil's claw (*Harpagophytum procumbens*) tuber

Blood Sugar StabiliTea

This tea helps stabilize blood sugar levels and can benefit those suffering from hypoglycemia as well as those with diabetes.

INFUSE

- 1 part blueberry (*Vaccinium* species) leaf
- ½ part fennel (*Foeniculum vulgare*) seed
- 1 part fenugreek (*Trigonella foenum-graecum*) seed

DECOCT

- 1 part dandelion root

Freshen-Bad-Breath Tea

Sweeten your breath with these mouth-freshening herbs!

INFUSE

- 1 part dandelion leaf
- 1 part peppermint (*Mentha × piperita*) leaf
- ½ part cardamom (*Elettaria cardamomum*) seeds, crushed

DECOCT

- 1 part Ceylon cinnamon (*Cinnamomum* species) chips

I'm-Sick-of-Cellulite Tea

Help your body metabolize fats and improve elimination of wastes with these cleansing herbs.

INFUSE

1 part dandelion leaf
1 part nettle (*Urtica dioica*) leaf

DECOCT

1 part dandelion root
1 part burdock (*Arctium lappa*) root

Children's Feel-Better Tea

These herbs can help the body fight infection and comfort the ailments of childhood, including colds, measles, mumps, and chicken pox.

INFUSE

1 part lemon balm (*Melissa officinalis*) herb
1 part anise (*Pimpinella anisum*) seed
1 part peppermint (*Mentha × piperita*) leaf

DECOCT

1 part dandelion root
1 part echinacea (*Echinacea purpurea*) root

Lower-Cholesterol Tea

This tea blend helps the body gradually break down
cholesterol and aids in its elimination.

INFUSE

1   part hawthorn (*Crataegus oxyacantha*) leaf,
flower, or berry

DECOCT

1   part dandelion root
1   part burdock (*Arctium lappa*) root
1   part ginger (*Zingiber officinale*) root

Clear-Skin Tea

By supporting the organs of elimination—the liver, kidneys,
and colon—these herbs encourage clearer skin, especially for
those suffering from acne, psoriasis, or eczema.

DECOCT

1   part dandelion root
1   part burdock (*Arctium lappa*) root
1   part yellow dock (*Rumex crispus*) root
1   part Oregon grape (*Mahonia repens*) root

Alleviate-Depression Tea

Liver cleansing, nerve nourishing, and mood elevating—consider these herbs when dealing with depression.

INFUSE

1   part St. John's wort (*Hypericum perforatum*) herb
1   part oat straw (*Avena sativa*) herb
1   part lemon balm (*Melissa officinalis*) herb

DECOCT

1   part dandelion root

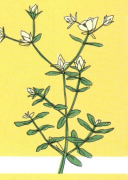

Decongestion Tea

This tea helps the body clear phlegm and open the lungs and sinuses.

INFUSE

1   part dandelion leaf
1   part nettle (*Urtica dioica*) herb
1   part thyme (*Thymus vulgaris*) herb

DECOCT

1   part dandelion root

Digestive Tea

When in need, reach for this multipurpose formula.
It can aid in the digestion of fats, prevent gas, and
soothe a stomachache.

INFUSE

1   part dandelion leaf
1   part peppermint (*Mentha × piperita*) leaf
½   part fennel (*Foeniculum vulgare*) seed

DECOCT

1   part dandelion root

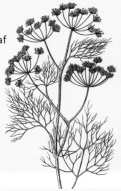

Edema Tea

This tea helps the kidneys eliminate excess fluid from the body.

INFUSE

1   part dandelion leaf
1   part nettle (*Urtica dioica*) leaf
1   part uva-ursi (*Arctostaphylos uva-ursi*) herb
1   part corn silk (*Zea mays*) stigma

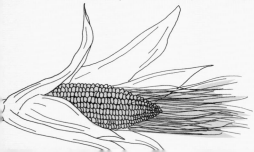

Increase-Energy Tea

Try this tea instead of coffee in the morning.
It's nourishing and mildly stimulating without the drawbacks
of addiction and the jitters.

INFUSE

1 part dandelion leaf
1 part yerba maté (*Ilex paraguariensis*) leaf
1 part nettle (*Urtica dioica*) leaf

DECOCT

1 part dandelion root

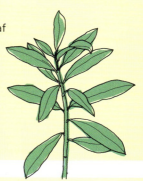

Fasting Tea

When you're fasting, drinking this tea will provide minerals,
improve your energy, and freshen your breath as well as
help cleanse metabolic wastes.

INFUSE

1 part nettle (*Urtica dioica*) leaf
1 part peppermint (*Mentha × piperita*) leaf
1 part fennel (*Foeniculum vulgare*) seed

DECOCT

1 part dandelion root

Headache Tea

This tea not only helps to relieve pain and stress but also helps reduce inflammation.

INFUSE

1 part German chamomile (*Matricaria recutita*) flower
1 part peppermint (*Mentha × piperita*) leaf

DECOCT

1 part dandelion root
1 part white willow (*Salix alba*) bark

Improve-Jaundice Tea

By improving liver function, these herbs help improve jaundice.

DECOCT

1 part dandelion root
1 part burdock (*Arctium lappa*) root
1 part Oregon grape (*Mahonia repens*) root
1 part yellow dock (*Rumex crispus*) root
½ part turmeric (*Curcuma longa*) powder or chopped root

Menopause-Relief Tea

These cool and calming herbs support
your hormones, build the blood, and help the liver
break down excessive hormones.

INFUSE

1 part vitex (*Vitex agnus-castus*) berry

DECOCT

1 part dandelion root
1 part black cohosh (*Actaea racemosa*) root
1 part dong quai (*Angelica sinensis*) root

Menstrual-Relief Tea

Rich in minerals, this blood-building tea improves liver
function so that hormones can be metabolized and reduces
stagnation in the breasts and reproductive system.

INFUSE

1 part dandelion leaf
1 part nettle (*Urtica dioica*) leaf
1 part red raspberry (*Rubus idaeus*) leaf

DECOCT

1 part dandelion root
1 part dong quai (*Angelica sinensis*) root

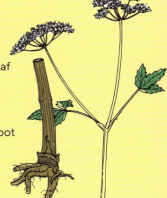

Mineral-Rich Tea

This herbal blend provides a wide variety of minerals.
It's exceptionally nourishing for the bones,
teeth, hair, and nails.

INFUSE

1 part dandelion leaf
1 part nettle (*Urtica dioica*) leaf
1 part horsetail (*Equisetum arvense*) herb
1 part oat straw (*Avena sativa*) herb

Nursing-Mother's Tea

This tea works to increase milk production and
improve milk's nutritional quality.

INFUSE

1 part dandelion leaf
1 part nettle (*Urtica dioica*) leaf
½ part fennel (*Foeniculum vulgare*) seed, crushed

DECOCT

1 part marsh mallow (*Althaea officinalis*) root

Pregnancy Tea

When you're pregnant, drink this nutritive tonic to tonify the uterus and help ease morning sickness.

INFUSE

- 1 part dandelion leaf
- 1 part red raspberry (*Rubus idaeus*) leaf
- 1 part nettle (*Urtica dioica*) leaf

DECOCT

- ½ part ginger (*Zingiber officinale*) root

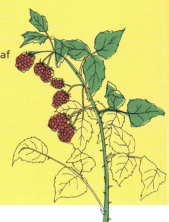

Prostate-Protection Tea

This tea improves circulation to the genitourinary system and reduces prostate inflammation.

INFUSE

- 1 part dandelion leaf
- 1 part nettle (*Urtica dioica*) leaf

DECOCT

- 1 part dandelion root
- 1 part saw palmetto (*Serenoa repens*) berry
- 1 part marsh mallow (*Althaea officinalis*) root

Sleep-Better Tea

Sleep better with these nerve-nourishing, calming herbs.

INFUSE

1 part dandelion leaf
1 part linden (*Tilia platyphyllos*) flower
1 part passionflower (*Passiflora incarnata*) herb

DECOCT

1 part kava (*Piper methysticum*) root

Postsurgery/Recovery Tea

This is an excellent blend for cleansing drug residue
out of the body and building strength and energy.

INFUSE

1 part dandelion leaf
1 part nettle (*Urtica dioica*) leaf

DECOCT

1 part dandelion root
½ part licorice (*Glycyrrhiza glabra*) root
1 part Siberian ginseng
   (*Eleutherococcus senticosus*) root

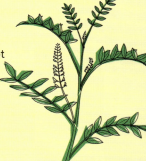

Swollen-Glands Tea

Try this blend for mumps, tonsillitis, and any glandular swelling. It works to improve lymphatic function.

INFUSE

1 part dandelion leaf
1 part cleavers (*Galium aparine*) herb

DECOCT

1 part dandelion root
1 part echinacea (*Echinacea purpurea*) root

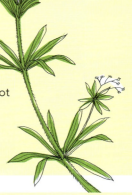

Urinary-Tract-Infection Tea

This tea is diuretic and soothing to inflammation in the urinary tract; it also helps fight infection.

INFUSE

1 part dandelion leaf
1 part uva-ursi (*Arctostaphylos uva-ursi*) herb
1 part corn silk (*Zea mays*) stigma
1 part buchu (*Agathosma* species) leaf

DECOCT

1 part marsh mallow (*Althaea officinalis*) root

Improve-Vision Tea

Improve your vision with the eye-nourishing herbs
in this blend. They provide beta-carotene and lutein and
increase circulation to the eyes.

INFUSE

- 1 part dandelion leaf
- 1 part dandelion flower
- ½ part bilberry (*Vaccinium myrtillus*) powder
- 1 part eyebright (*Euphrasia officinalis*) herb

DECOCT

- 1 part dandelion root

Vitamin C–Rich Tea

These vitamin C–rich herbs are also high in flavonoids, which
help improve the body's assimilation of that nutrient.

INFUSE

- 1 part dandelion leaf
- 1 part dog rose (*Rosa canina*) hip
- 1 part hibiscus (*Hibiscus rosa-sinensis*) flower
- 1 part red raspberry (*Rubus idaeus*) leaf

The-Weather-Is-Cold-and-I-Have-to-Be-Outside Tea

Warm yourself with the circulation-supporting
herbs in this blend.

DECOCT

1 part roasted dandelion root

1 part ginger (*Zingiber officinale*) root

1 part cinnamon (*Cinnamomum* species) bark

½ part licorice (*Glycyrrhiza glabra*) root

½ part prickly ash (*Zanthoxylum americanum*) bark

Weight-Loss Tea

Help the body metabolize fat, eliminate excess water, remain
energetic, and control its appetite with this blend.

INFUSE

1 part dandelion leaf

1 part nettle (*Urtica dioica*) leaf

1 part yerba maté (*Ilex paraguariensis*) leaf

1 part hawthorn (*Crataegus oxyacantha*)
leaf, flower, and/or berry

DECOCT

1 part dandelion root

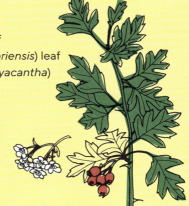

Making Juice

Dandelion leaves and roots can be put through a juicer to make a valuable tonic that helps counteract hyperacidity and normalizes the alkalinity of the system. It is rich in calcium, iron, magnesium, potassium, and sodium. The juice combines well with carrots and is used therapeutically for bone, spinal, and dental weakness.

Two cups of fresh leaves, run through a juicer, will make approximately ½ cup of juice. Store in the refrigerator. Take 1 to 6 tablespoons daily of this supremely nutritive tonic. Alternatively, combine ½ cup carrot juice, ½ cup dandelion juice, and ½ cup beet juice with the juice of 1 lemon or lime.

Juice Benefits for Specific Ailments

People with arthritis should take ½ cup of dandelion juice morning and evening on an empty stomach. The effectiveness of the juice is enhanced with a small amount of watercress juice. The juice is also recommended for the treatment of gout, obesity, hypertension, arteriosclerosis, Bright's disease, kidney stones, herpes, and night blindness (for the latter, make the juice from the flowers). As discussed in *Heinerman's Encyclopedia of Healing Juices*, S. Niedermeier, a German doctor, experimented with dandelion juice and found that it improved the eye disorders retinitis pigmentosa (atrophy of the inner layers of the eye's filtering system) and nyctalopeia (also known as night blindness).

There is also some indication that dandelion juice may treat tuberculosis: Its high beta-carotene content as well as its rich reserves of calcium and potassium salts can "strip" the bacteria from mucosal tissue in the lungs. Also, the lutein helps disinfect the lungs, so that bacteria have difficulty adhering to them.

Making Capsules

You can finely grind dandelion leaves and roots to go into capsules. (Pull-apart capsules are available from most natural foods stores and herb shops.) Powder the dried herb in a blender, a handful at a time, then fill both halves of the empty capsules and fit the halves together. Two dandelion capsules may be taken up to three times a day, as needed, for medicinal purposes.

Syrups

Syrups can be a delicious way to obtain the health and nutritional benefits of dandelions, and they can be taken daily or on occasion. They are an excellent method for persuading children to take herbal remedies. Syrups contain a lot of sugar, however, so use them in moderation.

Dandelion as a Homeopathic Remedy

The homeopathic dandelion remedy Taraxacum, available in most natural foods stores and herb shops, is made from an alcohol tincture of the entire plant before the flower opens. As in herbology, homeopathic usage of dandelion is for treating liver and digestive disorders. It is a remedy for ague, appetite loss, biliousness, debility, diabetes, flatulence (a feeling of bubbles in the bowels), gallstones, jaundice, liver, neuralgia, night sweats, rheumatism, a bitter taste in the mouth, an irritated tongue whose tissue is left raw and sore, and typhoid fever. It is used to treat frequent urination with difficulty in the passing of the urine and also extreme thirst. Taraxacum is usually given in a 1x or 3x potency.

Dandelion Spring Tonic Syrup

This spring tonic should be made with a variety of the spring herbs that grow wild in your area, such as dandelion leaves and roots, nettles, chickweed, and plantain. Because this recipe calls for brandy, pregnant women or alcohol-intolerant persons should avoid it.

Several handfuls of wild spring herbs (enough so the water just covers)

4 cups water

1 cup fruit juice concentrate

½ cup brandy

1. Chop the herbs and place in a pot. Add enough of the water to just cover the herbs. Bring to a boil, reduce the heat, and simmer until the liquid is reduced by half and is thick and dark-colored, which will take about 2 hours. Strain, reserving the liquid. You should have approximately 2 cups.

2. Mix in the fruit juice concentrate and the brandy. Pour into a glass container and store in the refrigerator. This syrup will keep for several months.

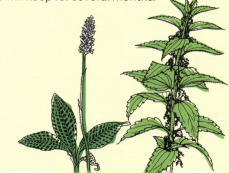

Dandelion Flower Syrup

MAKES ABOUT 2 CUPS

Use as a spread on bread and butter as you would honey.

- 2 very large handfuls of dandelion flowers
- 1 quart cold water
- 5 cups unrefined sugar
- ½ lemon, including peel

1. Place the dandelions and water in a saucepan and bring to a boil. Remove from the heat, cover, and let steep overnight.

2. The next day, strain and press the flowers to extract the liquid; compost the spent flowers. Return the liquid to the pan. Add the sugar and lemon, peel and all. Bring to a boil, reduce the heat, and simmer for a couple of hours or until the mixture is of a syrup consistency.

3. Remove and compost the lemon and pour the syrup into a glass container. Store in the refrigerator and use within 2 weeks.

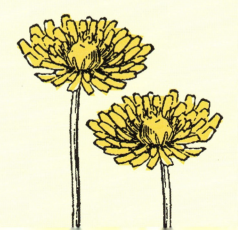

Delicious Dandelion Beverages

Dandelions can be prepared into a multitude of healthful, pleasant-tasting, nutrient-rich beverages beyond medicinal teas. Drinking dandelions may even alleviate some of the harmful effects of drinking too much coffee. Or enjoy dandelions in the traditional alcoholic forms of wine and beer, and as a cordial.

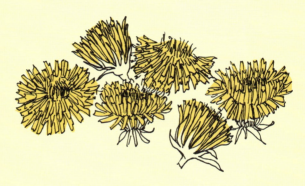

Giving Up Coffee for Good

Some people use the rich brew made from dandelion roots to extend their coffee and thus decrease the amount of caffeine they ingest. To give up coffee, gradually use less coffee and more dandelion root. By doing this over time, you can bypass the caffeine-withdrawal headache. Drinking dandelion root coffee helps diminish the craving for coffee flavor, as it has such a rich, earthy, roasted taste. Also consider dosages of the Overcoming-Addiction Tea (see page 88), which can strengthen both your willpower and your nerves.

DANDELION COFFEE

One of my favorite beverages is a dandelion "coffee" made from the dried and roasted roots. This drink tastes rich and earthy, similar to coffee, but without the caffeine. It is nonaddictive and much kinder to the stomach. Dandelion roots tend to be more bitter in summer and fall and sweeter in spring. Roasting dandelion roots releases aromatic compounds and converts the starch inulin into fructose, sweetening their taste.

Prepare the roots. Dig the roots (20 should give you enough for a small supply) in fall and wash well, using a vegetable brush to scrub them. Slice the roots lengthwise and allow them to dry in a warm place for 2 weeks.

Roast the dry roots. Preheat the oven to 200°F (95°C). Place the dry roots on a rimmed baking sheet and roast for 4 hours. (Alternatively, roast dried, sliced roots in a cast-iron skillet, stirring continually, about 20 minutes or until they are dark brown.) Cool completely before storing in a glass jar.

Brew. Simmer 1 heaping teaspoon of the roasted root in a cup of water, covered, for 10 minutes, then strain. The resulting dark, rich beverage will help you feel warmer. Alternatively, use the roasted roots as a coffee substitute by percolating them or brewing via the drip method.

Enjoy. Drink this as you would coffee, with cream and sugar or with honey and milk, as desired.

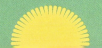

Warming Winter Spice Tea

MAKES 1 QUART

Slowly heat 4 cups of water in a pot. Put the following herbs
and spices into a mortar and with a pestle crush them slightly.
Alternatively, put them in a blender and pulse them briefly,
just enough to release some of the aromas.

DECOCT

- 2 parts roasted dandelion root
- ½ part cinnamon bark
- ½ part dried gingerroot
- ½ part decorticated (hulled) cardamom seeds
- ½ part star anise pod
- Honey to taste
- Milk or milk alternative to taste (optional)

Dandelion Mocktail

MAKES 2 OR 3 SERVINGS

- 100 small dandelion leaves
- 1½ cups tomato juice
- 2 tablespoons Worcestershire sauce
- A dash of hot sauce
- 2 or 3 celery stalks

Blend together the dandelion, tomato juice, Worcestershire,
and hot sauce. Pour into glasses and garnish each serving with
a celery stalk.

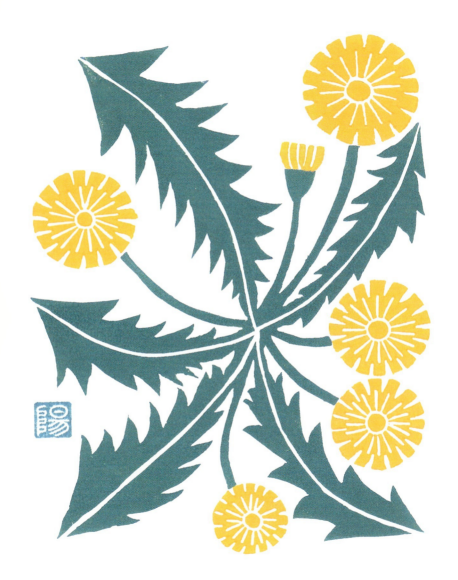

Dandelion Wine

Dandelion wine, believed to be of Celtic origin, is regarded as one of the fine country wines of Europe. In the late 1800s and early 1900s, it was not proper for ladies to drink alcohol; however, dandelion flower wine was considered so therapeutic to the kidneys and digestive system that it was deemed medicinal even for the ladies.

3	quarts dandelion blossoms, collected on a sunny day when fully open
1	gallon boiling water
2	oranges
1	lemon
3	pounds sugar
1	ounce active dry yeast
1	pound raisins

1. Remove any green parts on the dandelion blossoms; they will impair the fermentation.

2. Place the flowers in a large pot and pour the boiling water over them. Cover and let steep for 3 days.

3. Peel and juice the oranges and the lemon, saving the peels and reserving the liquid.

4. Add the orange and lemon peels to the flower-water mixture and bring to a boil. Remove from the heat, strain out the solids, then add the sugar, stirring until it is dissolved. Let cool to room temperature.

5. Stir in the orange and lemon juices, yeast, and raisins. Put everything into a crock with a loose lid (so gas can escape) to ferment.

6. When the mixture has stopped bubbling (after 2 to 7 days), fermentation is complete. Strain the liquid through several layers of cheesecloth and transfer to sterilized bottles. Slip a deflated balloon over the top of each bottle to monitor for further fermentation. When the balloon remains deflated for 24 hours, fermentation is complete. Cork the bottles and store in a cool, dark place for at least 6 months before drinking.

Dandelion Beer

During Victorian times in England, dandelion stout
was offered for sale.

1 quart fresh dandelion leaves (from young unflowered
plants) with some roots
1 gallon plus ¾ cup water
1 tablespoon active dry yeast (preservative-free)
1½ cups brown or unrefined sugar
1 tablespoon cream of tartar
Juice of ½ lemon

1. Place the dandelion leaves and roots in a large pot, add
1 gallon water, and bring to a boil. Reduce the heat, cover,
and simmer for 30 minutes. Remove from the heat and let
cool to room temperature, then strain.

2. In a small bowl, mix the yeast with the ¾ cup water and
1 tablespoon of the sugar. Cover and place in a warm area
for 10 minutes, until the mixture starts to foam. Pour it
into a large bowl, add the dandelion water, and stir in the
cream of tartar, lemon juice, and the remaining sugar.
Let sit for 30 minutes, then stir thoroughly.

3. Cover the bowl and keep at 65 to 70°F (18 to 21°C) for
12 to 24 hours, stirring occasionally with a wooden spoon,
until the mixture starts fizzing.

4. Transfer the liquid to sterilized bottles and leave them
out at room temperature for 3 hours, then refrigerate for
3 days. The beer will keep for 1 week. (If you have more
than you can drink in that amount of time, invite some
friends over to share this tasty brew!)

Dandelion Fizz

MAKES ABOUT 1 GALLON

5 cups dandelion flowers, stems removed
4½ quarts boiling water
4 cups sugar
2 lemons, sliced, with peel

1. Place the dandelion flowers in a crock and pour the boiling water over them. Cover and let stand for 12 hours.

2. Strain the dandelion water through several layers of cheesecloth into a large pot. Add the sugar and lemons. Heat gently to allow the sugar to dissolve, but not so much that the mixture boils, then remove from the heat.

3. Strain the liquid into sterilized bottles and let cool. Apply caps and store in a cool, dry place. After 3 to 4 weeks, the fizz will be ready to drink and should be stored in the refrigerator. It will keep for 3 to 4 months.

Dandelions are Nature's way of **giving dignity to weeds.**
—*Marvin, cartoon character*

Dandelion Cordial

MAKES ABOUT 1 QUART

3 cups dandelion flowers
1 quart vodka
⅔ cup honey
Zest of ½ lemon

1. Remove the dandelion petals from the green portions, but don't wash them; compost the green part.

2. Mix together the dandelion petals, vodka, honey, and lemon rind and pour into a widemouthed jar. Cap tightly and store in a cool, dry place for 2 weeks, shaking the jar every day.

3. Strain the ingredients through a fine-mesh strainer or several layers of cheesecloth. Discard the solids and rebottle the liquid. Drink it by itself or with a slice of lemon.

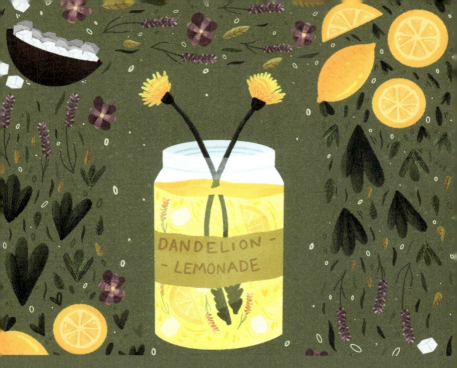

Dandelion Lemonade

Enjoy this sunshiny drink on a warm spring day!

MAKES 1 GALLON

4 cups dandelion flowers, rinsed

1 gallon spring water

1½ cups coconut sugar

Juice of 6 lemons

1. Soak dandelion flowers in water for 2 hours, then strain through a fine-mesh strainer or several layers of cheesecloth.

2. Stir the coconut sugar into the dandelion water until dissolved, then add the lemon juice.

3. Serve over ice with a slice of lemon.

Topical Medicinal Uses

Dandelion leaves are rich in chlorophyll, which speeds wound healing and helps prevent infection. The roots are cooling and can be used to help draw out and deter infections. Together, they could be prescribed for a number of specific health concerns.

Skin Irritations

Dandelion sap can be applied topically to bee stings, blisters, calluses, corns, and warts. The bitter white juice is most potent when the plant is in flower, in spring or summer—sap taken from plants in fall or winter will not be as effective. Just break open the stem or root and apply the sap to the area. Do this twice a day for five days.

Breast Health

Dandelion flower massage oil is recommended for breast massage. It helps release the negative emotions stored in the breast tissue and improves lymphatic movement. It is very helpful for those prone to breast cysts and lumps, and is a way of nurturing and giving positive attention to the breasts. You can also use a poultice of grated fresh roots or leaves to treat breast concerns such as cancer, cysts, and mastitis.

Fighting Infections

Use dandelion leaf as a bath herb to discourage yeast infections. Add a couple handfuls of the leaves to the bathwater. Run the water hot. Or place the leaves in a discarded sock and secure it with a hair tie to make cleanup easier—you'll still get the medicinal benefits in the tub. Dandelion leaf tea is also used as a wash in treating fungal infections.

Dandelion Massage Oil

The proportion of dandelion to olive oil isn't an important factor in making this massage oil. Simply keep in mind that the more blossoms you use, the more potent the oil. This is an excellent remedy to use for breast massage (see Breast Health, facing page) as well as to help skin heal. Collect the blossoms on a sunny, dry day in the morning, after the dew has evaporated.

> Dandelion flowers
> Dandelion roots
> Extra-virgin olive oil

INSTRUCTIONS

1. Spread the flowers on a screen and set them to dry in a cool, dry, shady, well-ventilated area for 2 to 3 days.

2. The day before you plan to make the oil, gather some dandelion roots. Wash them well and allow to dry overnight.

3. Chop the dried roots. Place the flowers and roots in a small glass jar. Cover with oil. Stir gently with a nonmetal utensil (such as a wooden chopstick) to force out any air bubbles, then top off with more oil. Seal and store in a cool, dry location at room temperature for 6 weeks.

4. Strain the infused oil through several layers of cheese-cloth. Discard the spent herb and rebottle and label the liquid. Refrigerated, the oil will keep for 3 to 4 months.

Dandelion Flower Essence

Dandelion flower essence, available from natural foods stores and herb shops, promotes relaxation and facilitates the release of negative emotions that are bound up in muscles, especially in the back, neck, and shoulders. It's an excellent flower essence to use when having bodywork, such as massage, done. And it's an excellent remedy for those who use their bodies a lot, such as massage therapists and athletes.

Dandelion flower essence also benefits those of us who overstructure our lives and find ourselves too busy to relax. It improves body-mind communication in tense people. It helps us let go of fear and have more trust in our ability to cope with life. By relaxing the physical body, it fosters spiritual openness and yet enables us to listen to and hear the messages of our body. It is used for people dealing with cancer or muscular degeneration, nervous people, and those with poor posture. It is also good for people who have a fear of being touched.

Cosmetic Uses

Dandelion has potential for cosmetic use. Because it is rich in emollients, it's useful in treating dry, sallow, and mature skins. Dandelion root tea is considered toning, meaning it helps invigorate the skin and brings out more beauty, and it can revitalize sallow skin. Or you can blend the leaves with a bit of water and apply the mixture to the face as a mask to brighten sallow skin. Add the leaves to facial steams and herbal baths to soothe and cleanse the skin.

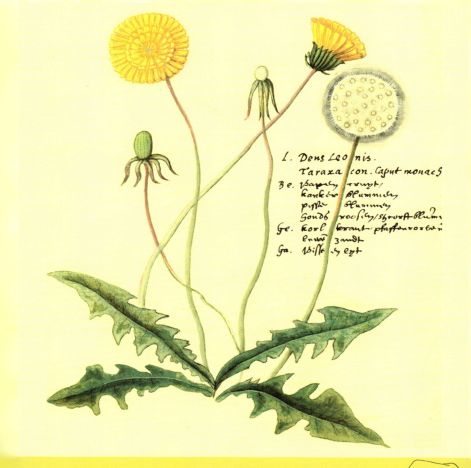

L. Dens Leonis.
Taraxacon. Caput monacᵉ
Be. Papely truyst/
kanker Blummen
pʸͭᵗ Blummen
Goudb roosken/shrout Blum?
Ge. korl kraut pfaffenrorlein
kruit zandt
Ga. Bille ᵍͭ eyt

Age Spots

Age spots, also known as brown spots or liver spots, usually
appear on the backs of the hands and are caused by the cumulative
effects of sunlight or chronic bruising of the skin. Fresh dandelion
sap, collected when the plant is in bloom in spring or summer,
can be applied directly to age spots to lighten them.

Herbal Bath

Adding dandelion to the bath helps remedy eczema and dry, oily, or itchy skin. It is also used as a bath herb for those who wish to lose weight.

2   cups boiling water
2   heaping teaspoons dried dandelion herb

1. Pour the boiling water over the dandelion in a bowl. Cover and let steep for 30 minutes.

2. Strain the infused tea and compost the spent herb. Add the tea to a full, warm bath, then get in for a soak!

Facial Steam

This gentle treatment will leave you with a fresh, radiant complexion.

2 cups water

2 heaping teaspoons dried dandelion leaves

1. Pour the water into a pot and bring to a boil. Remove from the heat, stir in the dandelion leaves, and set the hot pot on a table or countertop.

2. Sitting down at a comfortable height, position your head so that your face is about 10 inches away from the surface of the pot. Drape a towel over the pot and your head to contain the steam, and inhale the vapors and steam your facial skin for 5 minutes.

3. Rinse with a cold-water splash and pat dry.

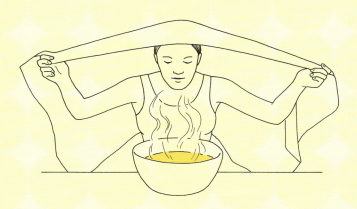

Dandelion Flower Water

MAKES ABOUT 1 CUP

In the 1800s, European women used dandelion flower water to lighten freckles, age spots, and small moles, and it's still used today to promote healthy, clear skin and prevent and treat blemishes.

1 cup freshly gathered, opened dandelion flowers
1½ cups water

1. Put the flowers and water in a pan and bring to a boil. Cover and simmer for 30 minutes.

2. Strain through a fine-mesh strainer or cheesecloth, squeezing the excess liquid out of the flowers, and store the flower water in a glass bottle in the refrigerator. Apply to the face with a cotton ball.

Dandelion Skin Oil

This facial oil softens the skin and helps disperse the congestion that contributes to breakouts.

4   medium-size fresh dandelion leaves
5   tablespoons castor oil

1. Wash, dry, and chop the dandelion leaves. Place them in a small pan with the castor oil and bring to a boil. Simmer for 10 minutes, then remove from the heat. Cover and let steep for 3 hours.

2. Strain the infused oil into a glass jar, and discard the spent herb. Store in the refrigerator. Apply to skin blemishes as necessary, using a clean cotton cloth or a cotton ball.

Dandelion Moisturizing Milk

MAKES ABOUT 1 CUP

This is both cleansing and moisturizing. It's excellent for improving sallow complexions.

½ cup boiling water

3 tablespoons elder flowers (*Sambucus canadensis* or *S. nigra*)

2 tablespoons dandelion leaves

½ cup milk

1. Pour the boiling water over the elder flowers and dandelion leaves in a bowl, stir, cover, and let steep for 12 hours.

2. Add the milk, stir well, and let steep for 2 hours. Strain into a glass container and store in the refrigerator. Apply gently to the face with a cotton ball.

Facial Wash

A dandelion facial is the perfect way to start your day!

2 cups boiling water
   A large handful of fresh-picked dandelion flowers

1. Pour the boiling water over the flowers in a bowl.
   Cover and let steep for 1 hour.

2. Strain to separate the flowers from the liquid,
   reserving both.

3. Apply the flowers (with some of the liquid) to the face
   and lie down for 10 minutes. Use the remaining liquid to
   rinse your face—no need to finish with water.

Dandelion Dye

MAKES 2 GALLONS

To make a light yellow dye for wool from the roots,
no mordant is required.

> 1 gallon chopped dandelion roots
> 1½ gallons water

1. Place the roots in a large pot and pour in the water. Allow to soak overnight.

2. Bring the mixture to a boil, reduce the heat, and simmer for 1 hour. Then strain and discard the spent roots.

3. Add enough cold water to make 2 gallons of liquid. Bring to a boil, add wet wool, reduce the heat, and simmer for 1 hour.

4. Rinse and dry the wool.

OTHER PRACTICAL USES

Dandelion has served humanity in diverse ways.
Not only can it feed, nourish, and enhance beauty, it can bring
color and comfort into our lives.

As a dye plant, dandelion root turns wool magenta
when alum is used as a mordant (fixative), purple when
tin and vinegar are used, and yellow when no mordant is added.
The flowers yield a **yellow dye**.

During World War II, the **latex sap** from the root of the
Russian dandelion (*Taraxacum kok-saghyz*), which is said to yield
four times the latex of other species, was used to make rubber.

When dandelions are dried and mixed with **potpourri**,
they add bulk and color (though not much aroma).

There are reports of dandelion leaves being dried and used as a
smoking mixture to help **asthma**. The leaves are combined
with equal parts of mullein (*Verbascum thapsus*) and rosemary
(*Rosmarinus officinalis*) and smoked very slowly in a waterpipe.

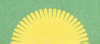

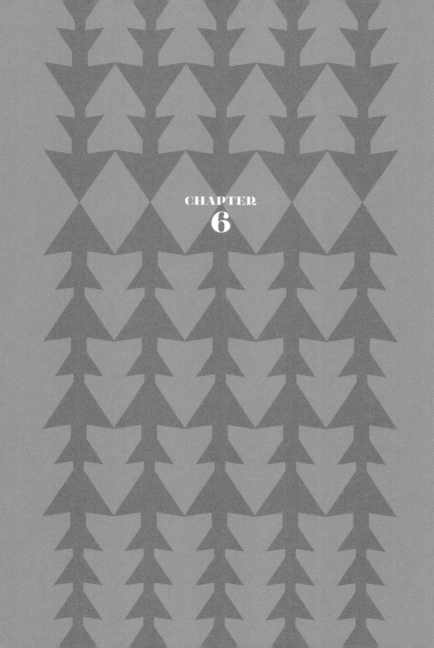

CHAPTER
6

Cooking with DANDELIONS

Dandelions provide a multitude of culinary possibilities. The young leaves are most commonly used; they should be gathered before the flower stalk achieves full height and before the flowers have yet formed. Try adding them raw to salads or in place of lettuce on sandwiches. Add them to cooked dishes such as soups, rice dishes, stir-fries, and omelets. Try juicing the fresh leaves and roots with carrots and spinach for a nutrient-rich beverage. You can also substitute dandelion greens in most recipes that call for spinach.

Notes on Preparation

Young dandelion flowers have a sweet, honeylike flavor; they get a bit more bitter as they age. Pick the flowers immediately before using so that they won't close up. Keep in mind that the green sepals attached to the flowers can be somewhat tart—great for some recipes, undesirable for others.

Consider how much time has likely passed since supermarket produce was picked, and from how many miles away it was transported. Now think about how wonderful it is to use something free, fresh, and local!

Preparing the Leaves

Old herbals report that it is better to wash and shred the leaves by hand rather than cut them with a knife. When the leaves are cut, cells are torn, and that releases an enzyme called ascorbic acid oxidase, which depletes vitamin C. It is always best to shred the leaves right before they are going to be used, to help conserve nutrients.

Cooking the Leaves

You can eat young leaves raw, but as they get older they are more palatable cooked. The French soak the leaves in salted water for half an hour to remove bitterness, although this does somewhat decrease the nutritional value. Even after the leaves become bitter, I still add them to certain dishes, as a little bitterness stimulates digestive secretions. However, you can minimize the sharp taste by cooking first in two changes of salted water or by adding a small amount of vinegar to the finished dish. After the first frost in autumn, the bitterness is dispersed and the leaves can easily be enjoyed again.

The best-tasting leaves are usually gathered from the center of plants growing in shady areas.

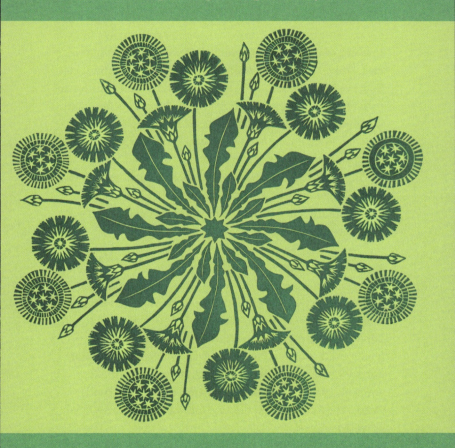

One pound of fresh greens
equals 2 quarts, and when cooked yields
1½ to 2 cups of cooked greens.

The chlorophyll content of dandelion leaves is sensitive to acids. When the leaves are cooked, the chlorophyll reacts with natural acids in the cooking water. A reaction with the carotene pigments causes a brown compound called pheophytin to form. To prevent the chlorophyll from reacting with any acids, leave the lid off the pot when cooking so that the acids may evaporate, or steam the plant quickly so there is little time for a reaction to occur. One other method is to cook the plant in plenty of water so that the acids are diluted. If you do this, though, do what wise Italians suggest: Drink the leftover water, which is said to beautify appearance.

Boiling dandelions will deplete some of their nutritional value, so steaming and stir-frying are the best methods of cooking. Basil, onion, lemon peel, and oregano pair well with dandelion leaf dishes.

Edible Flowers

Flowers are the colorful and fragrant sex organs of plants. They add grace and beauty, color, texture, and energizing pollen (which is the sperm of flowers) to one's diet. Because I don't want to rinse out the pollen, I pick just the clean blossoms. If you must clean them, simply rinse quickly and pat dry with a clean towel and keep refrigerated until they are ready to use. (Make sure there are no insects present.) Collect the flowers when they are fully opened, but not faded or wilted.

Remove their green calyxes. It is best to break up large blossoms by pulling off the petals and scattering them over a dish. Use them to garnish drinks, to float on top of a soup or in a punch bowl, or to embellish desserts.

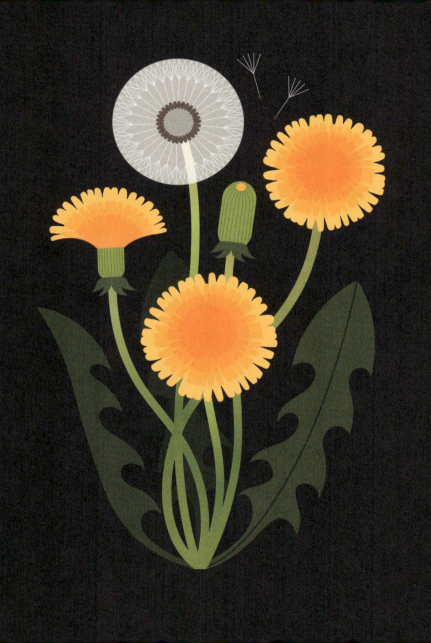

Nutritional and Healthful Constituents

Dandelion is considered one of the five most nutritious vegetables on Earth. Popeye may have gotten strength from spinach, but dandelion has twice the vitamin B_1 of that vegetable and six times the iron and four times the B_2 of iceberg lettuce. It contains 40 percent more vitamin C than tomatoes, 20 percent more beta-carotene than carrots, and more calcium than milk. One hundred grams of dandelion leaves provides 14,000 IU of provitamin A, whereas carrots provide 11,000. At only 45 calories per 100 grams, these generous greens are also a rich source of iron, manganese, and phosphorus. Choline, the member of the B complex that helps prevent fat buildup in the liver, is also present.

As every health-conscious individual knows, good nutrition is the most important part of good health. As evidenced by the lengthy lists that follow, not only does dandelion contain most of the vitamins and minerals recommended for a healthy diet—the ones you'll see called out in the nutritional information posted on the label of any packaged food—but it's also packed with a dizzying range of enzymes, acids, sugars, and other substances that nourish the health and energy of your entire body and all its systems.

The inulin present in dandelion root is currently under study for its potential as an immunostimulant as well as an aid for the kidneys and pancreas. Inulin is digested not in the stomach but, rather, in the colon by naturally occurring bacteria. Inulin encourages the growth of healthy intestinal flora. In a study conducted in 1995 at Dunn Clinical Nutrition Centre in Cambridge, England, eight subjects were given 15 grams of extra sugar daily for 15 days to feed unfriendly bacteria, such as *Candida albicans*, then given 15 grams of inulin for 15 days (about the amount in 2 ounces of fresh dandelion root). Results showed that the inulin increased a beneficial bacteria in the colon called bifidobacteria, which led to the conclusion that inulin could help improve the microflora of the intestines.

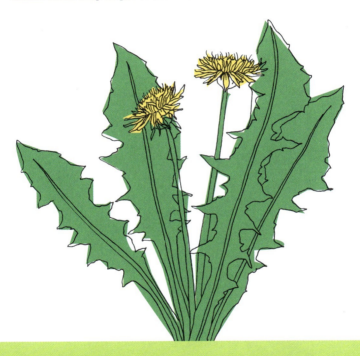

Dandelion greens are so good for you that you would do well to dry and powder them and place the powder in a saltshaker to be sprinkled on all your food as a nutritional supplement.

EAT MORE WILD GREENS!

Weeds are hardy. They grow easily, have survived centuries of adversity, and are often much more durable than our cultivated plants. Weeds often exist without any water except rainfall, are more resistant to frost and being trampled on, and offer themselves freely and abundantly. I love the fact that when I serve a wild salad or soup for dinner, most of the ingredients were growing just an hour earlier. It makes sense to learn to love and use them.

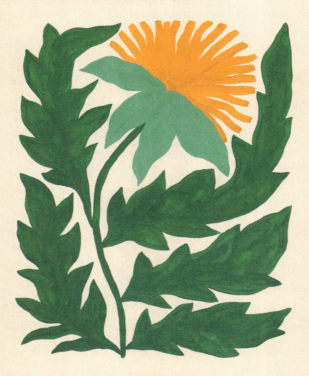

Here are a few ideas for how to prepare them, but also use your imagination to bring more green into your life!

Add to other greens to make a salad, or just eat the fresh greens on their own, simply dressed.

Rinse the greens well. Put them in a pan with ¼ cup of water and a few dashes of tamari. Cover and steam until tender.

Use greens as you would spinach in making lasagna.

Top greens with a mushroom sauce or a cream sauce.

Sauté greens with ginger and garlic and serve with rice. Or stir-fry with onions and curry powder, chili powder, Italian herbs, or Cajun spice blend.

Blend clean, chopped greens into low-fat yogurt, sour cream, or tofu. Season with lemon juice, garlic, salt, and sautéed chopped onion to make a dip.

Scramble eggs or tofu with greens. Here's your chance to have green eggs that would make Dr. Seuss proud!

Sauté greens with garlic, tomatoes, onion, and green bell pepper and serve with polenta.

Use greens as a filling for crêpes or in a soufflé.

Use raw wild greens in place of lettuce in sandwiches.

Make a loaf with greens, leftover cooked rice, sautéed onions, and sunflower seeds. Bake at 350°F (180°C) for ½ hour.

What the Root Contains

CONSTITUENT	NATURE/BENEFIT
Asparagine	Acts as a natural diuretic.
Caffeic acid	Helps treat allergies due to its anti-inflammatory properties.
Calcium	Nourishes bones, teeth, and nerves.
Choline	Helps metabolize fats and aids nerve and brain transmissions.
Coumestrol	Serves as a phytoestrogenic substance.
Essential oil	Contains antimicrobial properties.
Fatty acids (myristic, palmitic, stearic, lauric)	Benefit the nervous system and aid fat metabolism and digestion.
Flavonoid glycosides (apigenin and luteolin)	Exhibit diuretic, antispasmodic, antioxidant, and hepatoprotective properties.
Flavonoids (lutein, flavoxanthin, violaxanthin)	Serve as natural antioxidants.
Fructose	Is a fruit sugar.
Gallic acid	Tones tissues due to its astringent properties.
Hydroxyphenylacetic acid	Serves as a natural antioxidant.
Hydroxyphenylacetic gum	Soothes inflammation.
Hydroxyphenylacetic resin	Is naturally antiseptic.
Inulin	Helps keep blood sugar levels stable. The content is highest in autumn, up to 24 percent.
Iron	Builds the blood.
Lactucopicrin (bitter principle)	Stimulates natural digestive secretions.
Levulin	Is a starch, most concentrated in spring roots.
Mucilage	Soothes irritation.

CONSTITUENT	NATURE/BENEFIT
Pectin (soluble fiber)	May contribute to the plant's detoxifying abilities. In Russia, pectin is recommended to help the body detoxify from heavy metals and radioactivity.
Phenolic acids (including quinic acid and chlorogenic acid)	Contain antimicrobial properties.
Phosphorus	Benefits the heart and brain.
Polysaccharides (glucans, mannans, inulin)	Stimulate the immune system and benefit white blood cell production.
Potassium	Supports the kidneys and heart; dandelions contain about three times the potassium of most other greens.
Tannin	Restores tissue tone.
Taraxacerin	Is a crystalline, bitter substance.
Taraxacin	Is a bitter amorphous principle (root and leaves).
Triterpenes (taraxol, taraxerol, taraxasterol, amyrin)	May play a role in dandelion's liver- and bile-stimulating properties.*
Zinc	Supports the immune system.

***NOTE:** Taraxacin and taraxacerin are both actually combinations of triterpenoids and sterols (sitosterin, stigmasterin, phytosterin). These steroids have a structure similar to bile.

What the Leaves Contain

CONSTITUENT	NATURE/BENEFIT
Boron	Necessary for calcium metabolism and bone health.
Calcium lactate mannite	Builds healthy bones and teeth and supports heart function.
Chlorophyll	Helps cleanse bile from the blood and improves blood quality; helps the body utilize oxygen, prevents infection, and speeds wound healing.
Choline	As a component of lecithin, helps improve memory, nourish the nervous system, and prevent fat buildup in the liver.
Coumarin	Improves blood circulation.
Eudesmannolide	May play a part in dandelion's diuretic properties.
Fatty acids (linoleic and linolenic)	Assist in prostaglandin production, aiding immune response and reducing inflammatory conditions.
Flavonoid glycosides (apigenin and luteolin)	Improve circulation.
Folic acid	Builds the blood and helps prevent birth defects.
Germacranolide	May play a part in dandelion's diuretic properties.
Inositol	Helps nourish the brain and nervous system.
Iron	Builds the blood.
Lecithin	Helps fat metabolism and nourishes the brain, nervous system, and heart.
Nicotinic acid	Improves circulation and aids fat metabolism.
Potassium	Strengthens cardiovascular function.
Sesquiterpene lactones	Includes lactucin, lactucopikrin, and taraxacoside; antispasmodic, sedative, and anti-inflammatory properties.
Silica	Helps rebuild connective tissue and nourishes bones, hair, teeth, and nails.
Terpenoids	Act as nerve nutrients.

CONSTITUENT	NATURE/BENEFIT
Vitamin A	Strengthens mucous membranes and helps prevent infection; 100 grams of leaves contain 14,000 IU of vitamin A (more than carrots!).
Vitamin B	Supports the nervous system.
Vitamin C	Improves immune function and is necessary for collagen production.
Vitamin D	Assists in building healthy skin and bones.

What the Flowers Contain

CONSTITUENT	NATURE/BENEFIT
Carotenoids (taraxanthin, which is actually a mixture of lutein, flavoxanthin, violaxanthin, and chrysanthemaxanthin)	Strengthen the mucous membranes, boost the immune system, and are antioxidant (lutein is also especially beneficial for the eyes).
Lecithin	Nourishes the brain and nervous system and enhances fat metabolism.

What the Sap Contains

CONSTITUENT	NATURE/BENEFIT
Ceryl alcohol, tartaric acid, glycerin, caoutchouc, ester of acetic acids	Show a mild effect against candida.

Nutritional Value

100 grams (3.53 ounces) of raw dandelion leaves yields the following:

	RAW	COOKED
Calories	45	33
Protein	2.7 g	2 g
Fat	0.7 g	0.6 g
Carbohydrate	9.2 g	6.4 g
Fiber	1.6 g	1.3 g
Calcium	187 mg	140 mg
Phosphorus	66 mg	42 mg
Iron	3.1 mg	1.8 mg
Sodium	76 mg	44 mg
Magnesium	284 mg	171 mg
Potassium	397 mg	232 mg
Vitamin A	14,000 IU	11,700 IU
Thiamin	0.19 mg	0.13 mg
Riboflavin	0.26 mg	0.16 mg
Vitamin C	35 mg	18 mg
Water	85.6%	89.2%

DANDELION RECIPES

If the multitude of healthful and nutritional constituents of dandelion blossoms, leaves, sap, and roots hasn't yet convinced you that dandelion is one of nature's best foods, try the following recipes! I encourage you to use only the best ingredients—those that are organic, from pasture-raised animals, and preservative free.

BREAK YOUR FAST, HEALTHY AND FAST

Starting your day with healthy
fare sets the pace for the
rest of the day.

Green Eggs (or Tofu), No Ham

MAKES 3 SERVINGS

- 2 tablespoons coconut oil
- 2 cups chopped young dandelion leaves
- 6 eggs or a 14-ounce block of tofu
- 2 tablespoons milk or milk substitute
- ¼ teaspoon medium grind sea salt
- ¼ teaspoon freshly ground black pepper

1. Heat the oil in a skillet over medium heat.

2. Add the dandelion greens and stir until cooked, about
   10 minutes. Whisk the eggs, milk, salt, and pepper in a bowl;
   pour over the greens; and heat until the eggs are cooked,
   5 minutes or less. (Alternatively, whiz the greens, eggs, milk,
   salt, and pepper together in a blender, then cook the mixture
   in the skillet.)

Dandelion Buds with Eggs (or Tofu)

MAKES 2 SERVINGS

- 1 tablespoon vegetable oil
- 20 unopened dandelion flower buds
- 4 eggs or a 14-ounce block of tofu
- 1 tablespoon milk or milk substitute
- Sea salt to taste
- Freshly ground black pepper to taste
- Crisp toast, for serving

1. Heat the oil in a skillet over medium heat. Add the flower buds and stir until they start opening.

2. Mix in the eggs and milk, stirring gently with a fork, for 5 minutes, or until cooked to your liking. Season with salt and pepper and serve with toast.

Dandelion Florentine

MAKES 4 SERVINGS

- 4 cups chopped dandelion leaves
- 3 tablespoons cream cheese or vegan cream cheese
- 4 eggs
- ½ teaspoon medium grind sea salt
- Freshly ground black pepper to taste
- 4 slices whole-grain or gluten-free bread, toasted
- Salsa, for serving (optional)

1. In a skillet over medium heat, stir the dandelion greens and cream cheese for about 3 minutes.

2. Make four little indentations in the greens and nestle an egg in each spot. Cover and cook until the eggs are cooked to your liking, about 5 minutes.

3. Season with salt and pepper. Serve with a slice of toast and top with salsa, if you like.

Fruit Whip

MAKES 2 SERVINGS

1 banana, cut into chunks
1 apple, seeded and cut into chunks
1 avocado, cut into chunks
½ lemon with peel, seeds removed
1 cup young dandelion leaves

Combine the banana, apple, avocado, lemon with peel, and dandelion greens in a blender, adding enough water to reach a thick, blended pudding consistency.

Dandelion Flower Pancakes

MAKES 4 TO 6 PANCAKES

1 cup whole-wheat flour or gluten-free pancake blend
½ cup unbleached all-purpose flour or almond flour
1½ teaspoons baking soda
¼ teaspoon medium grind sea salt
1½ cups milk or milk substitute
1 egg, or 1 tablespoon chia seeds soaked in 2 tablespoons water
⅔ cup dandelion flowers, green portions removed
2 tablespoons coconut oil
Butter or vegan butter and maple syrup, for serving

1. Mix together the flours, baking soda, and salt in a medium bowl.

2. In a separate bowl, beat together the milk and egg, then stir into the dry ingredients. Add the flowers and stir.

3. Add the oil to a frying pan and drop the pancake batter by spoonfuls. When the edges just start to brown, flip and cook on the other side.

4. Serve with butter and maple syrup.

Dandelion Flower Waffles

MAKES 4 WAFFLES

1½ to 2	cups water
¾	cup rolled oats
¾	cup yellow cornmeal
½	cup dandelion petals
1	tablespoon vanilla extract
1	tablespoon vegetable oil, plus more for the waffle iron
¼	teaspoon medium grind sea salt
	Butter or vegan butter and maple syrup, for serving

Combine the water, oats, cornmeal, dandelion flowers, vanilla, oil, and salt in a large bowl. Ladle onto a hot greased waffle iron and cook until the waffle is nicely browned. Repeat with the remaining batter. Serve with butter and maple syrup.

Dandelion Popovers

MAKES 12 POPOVERS

2	cups chopped young dandelion leaves
4	eggs
1	cup unbleached all-purpose flour
1	cup milk or milk substitute
4	tablespoons softened butter or coconut oil, plus butter at room temperature, for serving
½	teaspoon medium grind sea salt

1. Preheat the oven to 375°F (190°C). Grease the wells of a muffin pan and place the pan in the oven to get hot.

2. Whiz together the dandelion greens, eggs, flour, milk, softened butter, and salt in a blender. Remove the hot muffin pan from the oven and fill the wells with the mixture. Bake for 35 minutes, until puffed and golden on top. Serve with butter.

DANDELION SALADS

Why drive to buy lettuce imported from another state that was in the ground weeks ago when you can harvest the fresh, free treasure in your yard?

Simple Dandelion Salad

MAKES 4 SERVINGS

- 3 cups young dandelion leaves from plants that haven't bloomed
- 10 dandelion flowers, freshly picked and washed, green portions removed
   Salad dressing, such as Simple Dressing (recipe follows)

Combine the leaves and flowers in a salad bowl. Add your favorite salad dressing just before serving.

Simple Dressing

MAKES 4 SERVINGS

- 3 tablespoons extra-virgin olive oil
- 1 tablespoon tamari or soy sauce
- 1 teaspoon raw apple cider vinegar

Whisk together the oil, tamari, and vinegar in a small bowl; serve immediately.

Dandelion Greens and Vinegar

MAKES 2 SERVINGS

- 5 cups chopped dandelion leaves
- 2 tablespoons raw apple cider vinegar
- 2 tablespoons extra-virgin olive oil
- 1 teaspoon chili powder or 2 tablespoons finely chopped fresh garden herb of your choice (thyme, rosemary, mint, etc.) (optional)
- ¼ teaspoon medium grind sea salt
  Nuts or edible flowers, for garnish

Place the dandelion greens in a bowl. With clean hands, thoroughly massage the vinegar, oil, chili powder (if using), and salt into the greens. Decorate the salad with nuts or flowers.

Mediterranean Salad

MAKES 4 SERVINGS AS AN APPETIZER, 2 SERVINGS AS AN ENTRÉE

- 4 tomatoes, chopped
- 2 cucumbers, chopped
- 1 cup chopped dandelion leaves
- ½ cup chopped fresh basil
- ¼ cup extra-virgin olive oil
- ¼ cup pitted sun-cured olives
- ½ teaspoon medium grind sea salt
  Juice of 2 lemons

Toss together all the ingredients in a large bowl.

Dandelion Salad with Cottage Cheese and Pecans

MAKES 4 SERVINGS

- ¼ cup chopped pecans
- 2 cups shredded young dandelion leaves
- 1 tomato, chopped
- 1 tablespoon chopped fresh parsley
- ½ cup cottage cheese
- 2 tablespoons olive oil
- 2 teaspoons tamari or soy sauce
- 1 teaspoon lemon juice or raw apple cider vinegar

1. Place the nuts on a tray and toast them in the toaster oven for about 3 minutes.

2. Arrange the dandelion greens, tomato, parsley, cottage cheese, and nuts in a salad bowl.

3. Toss with the oil, tamari, and lemon juice just before serving.

Coleslaw

MAKES 4 SERVINGS

- ½ head red cabbage, shredded
- ½ head white cabbage, shredded
- 2 carrots, grated
- 1 cup finely chopped young dandelion leaves
- ½ cup extra-virgin olive oil
- ¼ cup lemon juice
  1-inch piece of fresh ginger
- 1 teaspoon dry mustard
- ½ teaspoon medium grind sea salt

1. Toss the cabbages and carrots in a pretty bowl.

2. Combine the dandelion greens, oil, lemon juice, ginger, mustard, and salt in a blender and blend until thoroughly mixed. Pour on top of the cabbage and carrot mixture and serve.

Sauerkraut with Dandelions

MAKES 8 SERVINGS

Sauerkraut supports healthful intestinal flora and provides vitamin C. In ancient times, seafarers ate it to prevent scurvy. This recipe calls for using a pickle press; I bought mine online.

- 1 head white cabbage
- 1 head purple cabbage
- 2 cups chopped young dandelion leaves
- 4 teaspoons medium grind sea salt
- 1 teaspoon caraway seed or dill seed (optional)

1. Grate the cabbages (a food processor makes this easy). Toss with the dandelion greens, salt, and caraway seed.

2. Place the mixture in a pickle press and apply pressure. Leave undisturbed for 2 weeks.

3. When you open the press, you may find mold on top of the sauerkraut; scrape off and discard it. Rinse the sauerkraut well in a colander.

4. Store in the refrigerator, where it will keep for 3 to 4 weeks.

MIXING IT UP

Other fare can be mixed into cabbage sauerkraut, including apples, beets, broccoli, carrots, cauliflower, celery, onion, and daikon radish. Sauerkraut also can be flavored with 1 tablespoon per batch of chopped basil, caraway seed, chile peppers, dill seed, garlic, ginger, dulse, or kelp.

Dandelion Green Soup

MAKES 6 TO 8 SERVINGS

- 1 tablespoon olive oil
- 1 onion, finely chopped
- 1 garlic clove, chopped
- 2 teaspoons curry powder
- 2 cups chopped potato
- 4 cups chopped dandelion leaves
- 1 quart water
- ½ teaspoon medium grind sea salt
  Freshly ground black pepper
  Tamari

1. Heat the oil in a soup pot over medium heat. Add the onion, garlic, and curry powder, and sauté, stirring constantly, until the onion is translucent. Add the potatoes and dandelion greens, and sauté 3 to 5 minutes.

2. Stir in the water and cook until the potatoes are tender, about 30 minutes. Remove from the heat and let cool for 10 minutes, then carefully transfer the hot soup to a blender and purée until smooth or somewhat chunky, as you prefer. (Alternatively, use an immersion blender in the soup pot.)

3. Return the soup to the pot to reheat. Season with the salt, pepper, and tamari, and serve hot.

Dandelion Green Gazpacho

- 2 cups dandelion leaves
- 4 ripe tomatoes, halved
- ½ teaspoon medium grind sea salt
- 1 avocado, cut into chunks, or 3 tablespoons olive oil
- 1 cup water
- ¼ cup fresh basil or cilantro
   Juice of 1 lemon

Place all the ingredients in a food processor and pulse until blended but slightly chunky.

Dandelion Dumplings

- 1 tablespoon coconut oil
- 1 onion, chopped
- 2 cups rolled oats or leftover cooked rice
- 2 cups chopped dandelion leaves
- 1 beaten egg, or 1 tablespoon chia seeds soaked in 2 tablespoons water
- ¼ teaspoon grated nutmeg
- 1 teaspoon dried sage leaves
   Unbleached all-purpose flour or gluten-free flour blend

1. Preheat the oven to 350°F (180°C). Oil a 9- by 9-inch baking dish.

2. Heat the oil in a skillet over medium heat. Sauté the onion until tender, about 4 minutes. Stir in the oats, dandelion greens, egg, nutmeg, and sage, then add just enough flour to make a sticky dough. Form into 12 dumplings.

3. Place the dumplings in the prepared baking dish and bake for 45 minutes, turning them every 15 minutes, until golden brown on all sides. Serve in your favorite soup.

Dips can be served with chips, raw vegetables, or healthy crackers; piled on as sandwich fillings; or used as toppings and spreads.

Dandelion Dip

MAKES 2 CUPS

- 1 cup plain whole-milk yogurt or vegan yogurt
- 1 cup mayonnaise or vegan mayonnaise
- 2 cups chopped young dandelion leaves
- ¼ cup chopped fresh parsley
- 2 garlic cloves
- ½ teaspoon prepared horseradish
  Juice of 1 lemon
- ½ teaspoon medium grind sea salt

Place all the ingredients in a blender and purée until smooth. Eat immediately or enjoy within a couple of days.

Dandelion Green Raita

MAKES 2 SERVINGS

- 1 cup chopped dandelion leaves
- 3 tablespoons plain whole-milk yogurt or vegan yogurt
- 1 tablespoon olive oil
- 1 teaspoon lemon juice
- 2 tablespoons chopped fresh spearmint leaves
- ½ teaspoon medium grind sea salt

Combine all the ingredients in a small bowl and toss gently.
Eat immediately or enjoy within a couple of days.

Dandelion Pesto

MAKES ABOUT 2½ CUPS

- 3 packed cups fresh basil leaves (or arugula, young catnip, chervil, cilantro, dill, fennel, lemon balm, marjoram, mint, oregano, parsley, rosemary, sage, savory, thyme, or tarragon)
- 1 cup dandelion leaves
- 5 garlic cloves
- 1 cup raw pine nuts or walnuts
- ¾ cup olive oil
- 1 teaspoon medium grind sea salt

Place all the ingredients in a blender, or a food processor,
and purée until smooth. Eat immediately or refrigerate and enjoy
within a couple of days.

Dandelion Sauce

MAKES ABOUT 2 CUPS

- ¼ cup olive oil
- 1 onion, chopped
- 3 cups chopped dandelion leaves
- ¼ teaspoon cayenne pepper
- ½ cup fresh cilantro or basil
- ½ cup water
- ½ teaspoon medium grind sea salt

Heat the oil in a skillet over medium heat. Add the onion and sauté until transparent, about 5 minutes. Add the dandelion greens, cayenne, cilantro, water, and salt, and simmer for 10 minutes. Purée in a blender. Serve over baked potatoes, rice, or a protein of your choice. Eat immediately or refrigerate and enjoy within a couple of days.

Dandelion Sandwich Spread

MAKES 1 CUP

- ½ cup dandelion leaves or flowers
- ½ cup almond butter
- 1 tablespoon miso
  Juice of 1 lemon
  Water, as needed

Mix the dandelion, almond butter, miso, and lemon juice together in a small bowl. Add water, if needed, ½ teaspoon at a time, until the mixture reaches a spreadable consistency.

Dandelion Marinade

Dandelion leaves
1 part apple cider vinegar
1 part olive oil

1. Pack a widemouthed jar with fresh-picked dandelion leaves.

2. Fill the jar to the top with a 50:50 mixture of apple cider vinegar and olive oil. The herbs must be completely submerged and the vinegar-oil filled to the top so that there are no air spaces in the jar.

3. Screw on a plastic lid, or place a piece of wax paper under a metal lid so that the vinegar doesn't corrode it. Store the jar in a cool, dark place and enjoy the marinade as a dressing for salads or side dishes. This will keep in the refrigerator for about 10 days.

Savory Herb Butter
MAKES 1 CUP

1 cup softened butter, vegan butter, or coconut oil
2 teaspoons fresh dandelion flowers, green portions removed
2 teaspoons finely chopped dandelion leaves
¼ teaspoon medium grind sea salt

Place the butter in a small bowl. Top with the dandelion flowers, leaves, and salt, then use a fork to thoroughly mix them into the butter. Use immediately, or cover tightly and refrigerate for up to 1 week.

Sweet Herb Butter

MAKES ABOUT 1 CUP

- 1 cup softened butter, vegan butter, or coconut oil
- 2 teaspoons chopped dandelion flowers, green portions removed
- ¼ cup honey
- 1½ teaspoons grated organic orange peel

Place the butter in a small bowl. Top with the dandelion flowers, honey, and orange peel, then use a fork to thoroughly mix them into the butter. Use immediately, or cover tightly and refrigerate for up to 1 week.

Dandelion Jelly

MAKES 4 TO 6 (½-PINT) JARS

- 6 cups rinsed dandelion flowers, stems and green portions removed
- 3 cups water
- ½ teaspoon orange extract
- 1 (1-ounce) box of pectin
- 4½ cups sugar

1. Place the dandelion flowers and water in a large pot and bring to a boil. Reduce the heat to a simmer for 3 minutes. Remove from the heat, strain the liquid into a 4-cup glass measuring cup, and discard or compost the plant material.

2. Measure 2⅔ cups of the liquid and return it to the pot. Stir in the orange extract and pectin. Bring to a boil, then add the sugar. Return to a boil, stirring constantly, until the sugar is dissolved. Remove from the heat.

3. Skim off any foam from the top. Pour the liquid into sterilized canning jars. Process in a water bath canner for 10 minutes, or keep refrigerated and use within 2 weeks.

Dandelion "Mushrooms"

MAKES 2 SERVINGS

- ½ cup unbleached all-purpose flour or gluten-free flour blend
- ¼ teaspoon medium grind sea salt
- 15 dandelion flowers, freshly picked and still moist from being washed
- 2 tablespoons coconut oil or butter

1. Combine the flour and salt in a wide, shallow bowl. Dredge the dandelion flowers in the mixture until well coated.

2. Heat the oil in a saucepan over medium heat. Add the coated flowers to the pan, turning to brown on all sides, 2 to 3 minutes per side. Serve hot.

Dandelion Greens or Roots Stir-Fry

½ cup walnuts
1 tablespoon olive oil
4 garlic cloves, minced
½ teaspoon grated fresh ginger
4 cups chopped dandelion leaves (still moist from being washed) or dandelion roots
1 tablespoon tamari

1. Preheat the oven to 350°F (180°C). Spread the walnuts in a single layer on a baking sheet and bake for 10 minutes. Set aside.

2. Heat the oil in a skillet over medium heat. Stir in the garlic and ginger. If using dandelion greens, add them and the tamari, cover the pan, and steam for 5 minutes, stirring occasionally. (Add a bit of water if the mixture is too dry.) If using roots, sauté them with the garlic and ginger for 5 minutes; add the tamari in the last minute.

3. Top the greens or roots with the toasted walnuts before serving.

Sweet-and-Sour Greens

MAKES 2 SERVINGS

4 cups young dandelion leaves
2 tablespoons honey
¼ teaspoon dry mustard
3 tablespoons raw apple cider vinegar
  Sea salt to taste
  Freshly ground black pepper to taste
3 hard-boiled eggs, sliced (optional)

1. Wash the dandelion greens well and pat dry. Place in a serving bowl.

2. Mix the honey, mustard, and vinegar in a small bowl and season with salt and pepper to taste. Pour over the greens and toss to coat. Garnish with the sliced eggs, if desired.

ways to prepare dandelion crowns

The crown—the portion between the leaf and the root—is white and tender and makes an excellent vegetable. Trim off the leaves and root (reserve them for another recipe) and scrub the crown well to remove dirt. Boil in two changes of water. Season with a bit of butter, salt, and pepper. Crowns make an excellent addition to omelets, or you could wash, chop, and add them raw to a salad. Another method of preparation is to steam until tender (about 4 minutes), then marinate in salad dressing and add to salads.

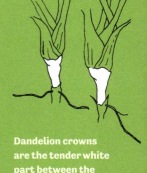

Dandelion crowns are the tender white part between the leaf and the root.

Dandelions Indian Style

MAKES 2 SERVINGS

½ teaspoon whole cumin seed
1 teaspoon whole coriander seed
1 teaspoon toasted sesame oil
4 cups chopped young dandelion leaves
½ cup water

Grind the cumin and coriander with a mortar and pestle or blender. Heat the oil in a large skillet over medium heat, then transfer the crushed seeds to the warm oil and stir for 3 minutes. Add the dandelion greens and water. Mix well. Cover and steam for 10 minutes.

Greek Dandelion Horta

MAKES 2 SERVINGS

15 dandelion leaves
1 small onion, chopped
8 black olives
2 tablespoons olive oil
1 tablespoon raw apple cider vinegar
Sea salt and freshly ground black pepper to taste

1. Add a few tablespoons of water to a skillet and steam the dandelion greens and onion until both are tender.

2. Add the olives, oil, vinegar, and salt and pepper to taste, and mix. Eat immediately or refrigerate and enjoy within a couple of days.

The star of our show can be local,
in season, abundant, healthful,
and delicious!

Dandelion Loaf

MAKES 6 SERVINGS

- 2 tablespoons vegetable oil
- 1 onion, chopped
- 1 celery stalk, chopped
- 1½ cups day-old bread pieces (approximately 1-inch pieces; can be gluten-free)
- 1 cup dandelion petals
- 2 eggs, or 2 tablespoons chia seeds soaked in 4 tablespoons water
- 1 tablespoon nutritional yeast
- 1 teaspoon chopped sage
- 1 teaspoon medium grind sea salt
- ½ teaspoon freshly ground black pepper
- 1 cup milk or milk substitute

1. Preheat the oven to 350°F (180°C). Grease a 9- by 9-inch baking dish.

2. Heat the oil in a skillet over medium heat. Add the onion and celery, and sauté until tender, about 5 minutes. Add the bread, dandelion flowers, eggs, nutritional yeast, sage, salt, and pepper. Mix well, then stir in the milk.

3. Pour the batter into the prepared baking dish and bake for 45 minutes, or until the top has browned. Slice and serve.

Dandelion-Potato Curry

MAKES 2 SERVINGS

- 1½ teaspoons coconut oil
- 2 garlic cloves, chopped
- 1 teaspoon curry powder
- 3 medium potatoes, cut into ½-inch cubes
- 4 cups chopped young dandelion leaves
- 2 cups water
- 1 teaspoon medium grind sea salt
- 2 tablespoons lemon juice

Heat the oil in a large saucepan over medium heat. Stir in the garlic and curry powder, and cook, stirring for 2 to 3 minutes. Add the potatoes, dandelion greens, and water. Stir, cover the pan, and cook for 15 minutes. Add the salt and lemon juice. Serve immediately or refrigerate and enjoy within a couple of days.

Dandelion Leaf Pizza

MAKES 1 SERVING

- 1 whole-wheat pita pocket
- ½ cup tomato sauce
- ¾ cup chopped dandelion leaves
- 2 slices mozzarella cheese or vegan mozzarella
- 1 teaspoon chopped fresh basil

Cover one side of the pita with the tomato sauce. Add the dandelion greens and top with the cheese. Broil in a toaster oven until the cheese melts, about 5 minutes. Top with the basil and serve immediately.

Dandelion Lasagna

MAKES 6 SERVINGS

- 1 tablespoon extra-virgin olive oil
- 3 garlic cloves
- 1 tablespoon chopped fresh parsley
- 1 tablespoon chopped fresh basil
- 1 tablespoon chopped fresh oregano
- 1 teaspoon fennel seed
- 6 cups chopped dandelion leaves
- 6 cups tomato sauce
- 6 ounces tomato paste
  Salt and pepper to taste
- 2 13-ounce boxes lasagna noodles (can be gluten-free)
- 2 cups ricotta cheese or vegan cheese

1. Preheat the oven to 375°F (190°C). Grease an 8- by 12-inch baking dish.

2. Heat the oil in a skillet over medium heat. Add the garlic, parsley, basil, oregano, and fennel seed, and sauté for a few minutes, until the garlic is cooked. Add the dandelion greens, still stirring, and cook until they are wilted. Add the tomato sauce, tomato paste, salt, and pepper. Simmer for 2 hours, stirring occasionally.

3. Bring 6 quarts water to a boil in a large pot. Drop in the lasagna noodles and cook until the pasta is tender, about 12 minutes. Drain.

4. Place a layer of noodles in the prepared baking dish and cover with half the sauce. Spread the cheese evenly over the sauce. Cover with another layer of noodles. Cover with the remaining sauce.

5. Bake for 30 minutes, until the cheese is nicely melted and the sauce is bubbly. Serve immediately.

Dandelion Greens with Pasta

MAKES 4 SERVINGS

- ¾ pound capellini or a gluten-free pasta of your choice
- 2 tablespoons butter or olive oil
- 5 cups chopped dandelion leaves
- 4 garlic cloves, chopped
- 2 tablespoons chopped fresh basil
- ½ cup nutritional yeast
- 3 tablespoons plain whole-milk yogurt or vegan yogurt
- ½ teaspoon grated nutmeg
- ½ teaspoon medium grind sea salt
- ½ teaspoon freshly ground black pepper

1. Bring 3 quarts water to a boil in a large pot, add the pasta, and cook until tender, about 12 minutes. Drain.

2. While the pasta is cooking, melt the butter in a large skillet over medium heat. Add the dandelion greens, garlic, and basil, and cook, stirring occasionally, for 5 minutes. Reduce the heat to low and add nutritional yeast, yogurt, nutmeg, salt, and pepper. Serve over the drained pasta.

Dandelion Polenta

MAKES 4 SERVINGS

- 1 cup cornmeal
- ¾ teaspoon medium grind sea salt
  Additions: fresh basil or cilantro, sun-dried tomatoes, pesto, chopped garlic, sautéed mushrooms (optional)
- ¾ cup chopped dandelion leaves
- ¾ cup grated provolone, fontina, or vegan cheese

Bring 4 cups water to a boil in a large saucepan. Add the cornmeal and salt, and stir well. Stir in any additions, if desired. Cook over low heat until the polenta thickens, about 15 minutes. Stir in the dandelion greens and cheese. Serve hot. Leftovers can be poured into an oiled baking dish, smoothed out, and later cut into squares and pan-fried.

Dandelion Spanakopita

MAKES 6 SERVINGS

- 3 tablespoons butter or olive oil
- 1 large onion, chopped
- 8 cups chopped young dandelion leaves
- 1 tablespoon chopped fresh basil
- 1 teaspoon chopped fresh oregano
- ½ teaspoon medium grind sea salt
- ¼ teaspoon freshly ground black pepper
- 1 box (16 ounces) frozen filo dough, thawed
- 1 cup (2 sticks) butter, melted, or 1 cup coconut oil
- 2 cups feta cheese, crumbled, or vegan feta

1. Preheat the oven to 350°F (180°C). Lightly grease a 9- by 13-inch baking dish.

2. Heat the 3 tablespoons butter in a skillet over medium heat. Add the onion and sauté until transparent, then add the dandelion greens, basil, oregano, salt, and pepper, and cook, stirring occasionally, for 5 minutes.

3. Place a filo dough leaf in the prepared baking dish and brush with some of the melted butter. Add seven more layers, brushing with melted butter between each layer. Spoon half of the sautéed dandelion mixture and half of the feta onto the filo. Add eight more layers of filo, brushing each layer with butter. Spoon the rest of the dandelion mixture and feta onto the filo, followed by eight more buttered layers of filo. Bake for 45 minutes, until golden brown on top.

Dandelion Greens Quiche

MAKES 1 (10-INCH) QUICHE

CRUST

- ½ cup extra-virgin olive oil
- 2 tablespoons milk or milk substitute
- ¾ cup unbleached all-purpose flour, ground walnuts, or gluten-free flour blend
- ¾ cup cornmeal
- 1 tablespoon chopped fresh sage
- ½ teaspoon medium grind sea salt
- ¼ teaspoon freshly ground black pepper

FILLING

- 1 tablespoon extra-virgin olive oil
- 1 medium onion, chopped
- 1 cup grated cheddar cheese or vegan cheese
- 2½ cups chopped dandelion leaves
- 2 eggs
- 1 teaspoon medium grind sea salt
- Freshly ground black pepper to taste

INSTRUCTIONS

1. Preheat the oven to 425°F (220°C).

2. Combine the oil and milk in a large mixing bowl. Add the flour, cornmeal, sage, salt, and pepper, and stir until a dough comes together.

3. Press the dough into a 10-inch pie pan. Bake for 5 to 7 minutes, until the edges are golden. Set aside. Reduce the oven temperature to 350°F (180°C).

4. Heat the oil in a skillet. Add the onion and lightly sauté it at medium heat until tender, about 5 minutes. Scrape it into the prebaked pie shell. Add the cheese and dandelion greens.

5. Whiz the eggs in a blender with salt and pepper to taste. Pour over the greens in the pie shell. Bake for 35 minutes, or until the quiche is browned on top and a knife inserted in the center comes out clean. Let stand for a few minutes before serving.

Irish Stew
MAKES 6 SERVINGS

- 1 tablespoon extra-virgin olive oil
- 2 onions, chopped
- 2 tablespoons chopped fresh thyme
- 1 tablespoon chopped fresh rosemary
- 1 pound lamb cubes or about 1½ cups cubed tempeh
- 2 potatoes, cubed
- 3 carrots, sliced
- 2 cups chopped dandelion leaves
- 2 cups water
- 1 8-ounce bag frozen peas
- 3 tablespoons unbleached all-purpose flour or gluten-free flour blend
- 1 teaspoon medium grind sea salt
- 1 teaspoon freshly ground black pepper

1. Heat the oil in a large pot over medium heat. Add the onions and sauté until translucent. Stir in the thyme and rosemary, then add the lamb, potatoes, carrots, and dandelion greens, stirring occasionally until the lamb is browned, about 10 minutes.

2. Stir in 2 cups water, peas, flour, salt, and pepper, and simmer for 1½ hours.

Roots to Get Grounded

MAKES 4 TO 6 SERVINGS

1 cup carrots, sliced into ¼-inch rounds

1 cup chopped onions

1 cup potatoes, cut into ½-inch cubes

1 cup sweet potatoes, peeled and cut into ½-inch cubes

½ cup rutabaga, peeled and cut into ¼-inch cubes

½ cup beets, peeled and cut into ¼-inch cubes

1 14-ounce package tempeh, sliced into 16 pieces

1 cup finely chopped dandelion roots

1 tablespoon extra-virgin olive oil

2 tablespoons red wine

2 tablespoons water

2 tablespoons tamari

2 garlic cloves, minced

1 tablespoon grated fresh ginger

1. Preheat the oven to 400°F (200°C).

2. Place all the ingredients into a baking dish that has a lid. Stir until everything is well mixed. Bake, covered, for 1 hour.

Carrot-Rice Loaf with Dandelion

MAKES 6 SERVINGS

1 tablespoon coconut oil

1 onion, chopped

4 cups grated raw carrots

4 cups cooked brown rice

½ cup almond butter

½ cup chopped dandelion leaves

½ cup coarse bread crumbs (can be gluten-free)

1 tablespoon chopped fresh sage

1 teaspoon medium grind sea salt

1. Preheat the oven to 350°F (180°C). Grease a 9- by 9-inch baking dish.

2. Heat the oil in a small skillet over medium heat. Add the onion and sauté until tender, about 5 minutes.

3. Mix the carrots, rice, almond butter, and dandelion greens in a large bowl. Stir in the sautéed onion, bread crumbs, sage, and salt, then scrape the mixture into the prepared baking dish. Bake for 45 minutes.

Dandelion Flower Burgers

MAKES 3 OR 4 BURGERS

3 tablespoons vegetable oil

½ cup chopped onion

1 cup packed dandelion flowers, stems and green portions removed

½ cup unbleached all-purpose flour or gluten-free flour blend

2 tablespoons milk or milk substitute

½ teaspoon dried or 1 teaspoon chopped fresh basil

½ teaspoon dried or 1 teaspoon chopped fresh sage

½ teaspoon medium grind sea salt

1. Heat half of the oil in a small skillet over medium heat. Add the onion and sauté until tender, about 5 minutes. Transfer the onion to a large bowl and add the dandelion flowers, flour, milk, basil, sage, and salt. Mix well, then form into patties.

2. Heat the remaining oil in a cast-iron skillet. When the oil is hot, fry the patties, flipping once, until golden brown, 3 to 5 minutes per side.

Dandelion Greens Patties

MAKES 6 PATTIES

- 3 cups mashed potatoes
- 2 cups chopped dandelion leaves
- 1 onion, chopped
- ½ cup raw sunflower seeds
- 3 tablespoons nutritional yeast
- 1 egg, or 1 tablespoon chia seeds soaked in 2 tablespoons water
- 1 teaspoon medium grind sea salt
- ¼ teaspoon chopped dried rosemary or ½ teaspoon fresh rosemary

1. Preheat the oven to 400°F (200°C). Grease a baking sheet.

2. Combine the potatoes, dandelion greens, onion, sunflower seeds, nutritional yeast, egg, salt, and rosemary in a large bowl. Shape the mixture into patties. Bake on the prepared sheet for 30 minutes, turning over after 15 minutes, until golden brown on each side.

Dandelion Soufflé

- 4 cups chopped young dandelion leaves
- 1 cup milk or milk substitute
- ¼ cup grated cheddar cheese or vegan cheese
- 3 tablespoons coconut oil
- 3 tablespoons unbleached all-purpose flour or gluten-free flour blend
- 3 tablespoons nutritional yeast
- ½ teaspoon grated nutmeg
- ¼ teaspoon medium grind sea salt
- 4 eggs, separated

1. Preheat the oven to 375°F (190°C). Grease six individual custard cups and place them on a baking sheet.

2. Put the dandelion greens, milk, cheese, oil, flour, nutritional yeast, nutmeg, salt, and egg yolks into a blender and purée. Using a hand or stand mixer, beat the egg whites until stiff peaks form and slowly mix into the blended dandelion mixture.

3. Pour the batter into the prepared custard cups. Slide the baking sheet with the cups into the oven and bake for 40 minutes, or until firm.

Dandelion-Potato Bake

MAKES 4 SERVINGS

- 3 tablespoons extra-virgin olive oil or butter
- 5 potatoes, thinly sliced
- 4 cups chopped young dandelion leaves
- 1 onion, sliced
- 1 teaspoon grated nutmeg
- 1 teaspoon dried rosemary
  Sea salt and freshly ground black pepper
- 2 cups milk or milk substitute

1. Preheat the oven to 350°F (180°C). Grease a 9- by 9-inch baking dish with the oil.

2. Layer the prepared baking dish with potato slices, dandelion greens, and onion slices. Sprinkle with the nutmeg, rosemary, and salt and pepper to taste. Pour the milk over the veggies, and bake for 1 hour.

Dandelions and Rice

MAKES 6 SERVINGS

- 3 tablespoons coconut or olive oil
- 1 large onion, chopped
- 4 cups chopped young dandelion leaves
- 4 cups cooked basmati rice, brown rice, or wild rice
- 1 teaspoon medium grind sea salt

Heat the oil in a skillet over medium heat and sauté the onion until transparent, about 5 minutes. Add the dandelion greens and stir occasionally for about 5 minutes. Mix in the rice and salt.

Dandelion Rice Balls

MAKES 12 BALLS

- 1 tablespoon coconut oil
- 1 onion, finely chopped
- 6 cups chopped young dandelion leaves
- 2 cups cooked basmati rice
- 3 tablespoons almond butter
- 1 tablespoon lemon juice
- 2 teaspoons chopped fresh dill weed
- 1 teaspoon medium grind sea salt
- ¼ teaspoon freshly ground black pepper
- 1 cup bread crumbs (can be gluten-free)

1. Preheat the oven to 350°F (180°C). Grease a baking sheet.

2. Heat the oil in a skillet over medium heat. Add the onion and sauté until tender, about 5 minutes. Transfer the onion to a large mixing bowl, then add the dandelion greens, rice, almond butter, lemon juice, dill, salt, and pepper, stirring well. With damp hands, form balls, using about ¼ cup of the mixture for each ball.

3. Place the bread crumbs in a shallow bowl. Roll each ball in the crumbs and place on the prepared baking sheet. Bake for 25 minutes, or until golden brown on all sides.

Dandelion Flower Muffins
MAKES ABOUT 12 MUFFINS

- ¼ cup coconut oil
- ½ cup coconut sugar
- 1 egg, or 1 tablespoon chia seeds soaked in 2 tablespoons water
- 1 tablespoon baking powder
- 2 teaspoons ground cinnamon
- ½ teaspoon medium grind sea salt
- 2 cups milk or milk substitute
- 3 cups unbleached all-purpose flour or gluten-free flour blend
- 1 cup cornmeal
- 1 cup dandelion flower petals (sepals removed)

1. Preheat the oven to 350°F (180°C). Grease 12 wells of one muffin pan.

2. Mix together the oil and sugar in a large bowl. Add the egg, baking powder, cinnamon, and salt, and combine thoroughly. Stir in the milk, flour, and cornmeal bit by bit, alternating wet and dry ingredients.

3. Add the dandelion petals and stir just to moisten all the ingredients; you don't want to overmix.

4. Spoon the batter into the prepared muffin wells and bake for 35 minutes, or until the tops are golden. Let cool for 10 minutes before attempting to remove the muffins from the pan.

Dandelion Biscuits

MAKES 12 TO 16 BISCUITS

- 1 cup whole-wheat flour or gluten-free flour blend, plus more for kneading
- ¾ cup cornmeal
- 2 teaspoons baking powder
- ¼ teaspoon medium grind sea salt
- ¾ cup plain whole-milk yogurt or vegan yogurt
- ½ cup dandelion flower petals (sepals removed)
- 2 tablespoons coconut oil

1. Preheat the oven to 425°F (220°C). Lightly oil a baking sheet.

2. Sift together the flour, cornmeal, baking powder, and salt into a large bowl. Add the yogurt, dandelion petals, and oil, and stir for 3 minutes.

3. Turn out the mixture onto a lightly floured board and roll it into a ball. Using a rolling pin, roll to a thickness of ¼ inch. Cut with a 2-inch biscuit cutter or a jar lid of similar diameter. Space the biscuits 2 inches apart on the prepared baking sheet.

4. Bake for 12 minutes, or until the biscuits are puffed up and golden.

Dandelion Bread

MAKES 1 LOAF

½ cup warm water (about 100°F [38°C])

1 tablespoon honey

2 tablespoons active dry yeast

1½ cups hot water (about 130°F [55°C])

1 cup cornmeal

2 tablespoons coconut oil

1½ teaspoons medium grind sea salt

2 cups whole-wheat flour

2 cups unbleached all-purpose flour, plus more for kneading

1 cup finely chopped dandelion leaves

1. Combine the warm water, honey, and yeast in a small bowl and let stand until the mixture foams up, 3 to 5 minutes. In a separate bowl, combine the hot water, cornmeal, oil, and salt. When the cornmeal mixture has cooled to lukewarm, stir in the yeast mixture. Then add the flours, 1 cup at a time. Stir in the dandelion greens. Knead on a lightly floured surface for 3 minutes. Place the dough in an oiled bowl, cover, and let rise in a warm place until tripled in size.

2. Preheat the oven to 450°F (230°C). Oil a loaf pan.

3. Beat down and shape the dough into a loaf and place it in the prepared loaf pan. Allow to rise for 15 minutes, then bake for 10 minutes. Reduce the oven temperature to 350°F (180°C) and bake for 50 minutes. Let cool on a rack for 5 to 10 minutes before removing from the pan.

DANDY DESSERTS

These desserts are—you guessed it!—
just dandy.

Dandy Lemon Pudding

MAKES 2 SERVINGS

1   cup Brazil nuts, soaked overnight
8   dates, soaked for 20 minutes
    Juice of 3 lemons
1   teaspoon grated lemon peel
2   tablespoons dandelion flowers, green portions
    removed and flowers petals separated

Drain the soaked nuts and dates, reserving the date liquid.
Combine the nuts, dates, lemon juice, lemon peel, and dandelion
flowers in a food processor and purée until well blended. Add a
bit of the date liquid, if needed, to reach a puddinglike consistency.
Pour into individual dishes and garnish with a dandelion flower.

Dandelion Pie

MAKES 8 SERVINGS

⅔ cup coconut sugar

4 egg yolks, or 4 tablespoons chia seeds soaked in
   8 tablespoons water

2 teaspoons grated lemon peel

2 tablespoons unbleached all-purpose flour or
   gluten-free flour blend

1½ cups milk or milk alternative

1 cup dandelion flowers, green portions removed

½ cup sunflower seeds

1 unbaked frozen piecrust

1. Preheat the oven to 350°F (180°C).

2. Mix together the coconut sugar, egg yolks, lemon peel,
   and flour in a saucepan. Slowly beat in the milk and
   cook over low heat, stirring until the custard thickens.
   Don't let the mixture scorch.

3. Pulverize the dandelion flowers in a food processor.
   Add to the custard mixture and stir in the sunflower seeds.
   Pour the batter into the piecrust and bake for 20 minutes,
   or until the top is browned and a knife inserted in the
   center comes out clean.

Dandelion Flower Cookies

MAKES 24 COOKIES

- ½ cup coconut oil
- ½ cup coconut sugar
- 2 eggs, or 2 tablespoons chia seeds soaked in 4 tablespoons water
- 1 teaspoon vanilla extract
- 1 cup unbleached all-purpose flour or gluten-free flour blend
- 1 cup quick or rolled oats, powdered in the blender
- ½ cup dandelion petals, green portions removed

Preheat the oven to 375°F (190°C). Grease a baking sheet. Combine all of the ingredients and drop the dough in balls onto the baking sheet, leaving an inch of space between them and flattening them slightly with a fork. Bake for 20 minutes or until golden brown.

Flower Frozen Pops

Here's a quick summer treat children are sure to love. Fill frozen pop molds with apple juice to which you've added the juice of 1 lime. Press a dandelion flower, green portions removed, into the center of each compartment. Freeze for at least 3 hours.

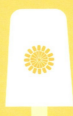

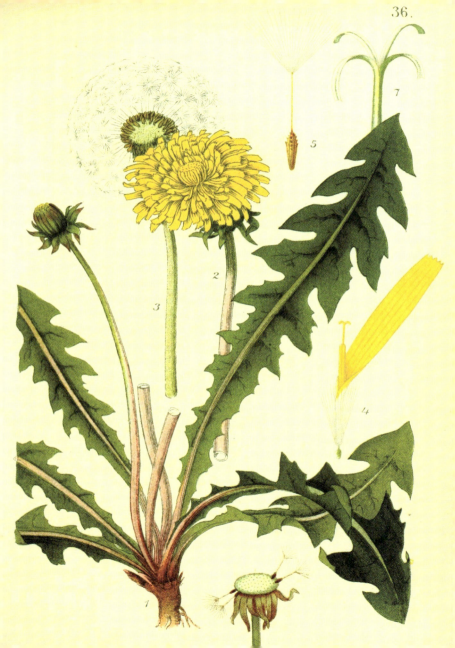

Converting to Metric Measurements

TEASPOONS TO MILLILITERS

¼ teaspoon = 1 ml
⅓ teaspoon = 2 ml
½ teaspoon = 2.5 ml
¾ teaspoon = 4 ml
1 teaspoon = 5 ml

TABLESPOONS TO MILLILITERS

¼ tablespoon = 4 ml
½ tablespoon = 8 ml
1 tablespoon = 15 ml

CUPS TO MILLILITERS

⅛ cup = 30 ml
¼ cup = 59 ml
⅓ cup = 79 ml
½ cup = 118 ml
⅔ cup = 150 ml
¾ cup = 180 ml
1 cup = 237 ml
2 cups = 473 ml = 1 pint

4 cups = 1 quart = 946 ml,
     or approximately 1 liter
4 quarts = 1 gallon = 4 liters

OUNCES TO GRAMS

¼ ounce = 7 g
⅓ ounce = 9.3 g
½ ounce = 14 g
1 ounce = 28 g
2 ounces = 56 g
3 ounces = 84 g
4 ounces = 112 g
6 ounces = 168 g
8 ounces = 224 g
16 ounces = 1 pound = 454 g
2.2 pounds = 1 kilogram

Resources

ORGANIC HERBS
Trout Lake Farm
https://troutlakefarm.com

FRESH AND DRIED HERBS

If you can't gather your own and don't have a local source, you can always obtain dried dandelion leaves and roots from mail-order herb shops such as those listed here.

Rebecca's Herbal Apothecary
https://rebeccasherbs.com

Mountain Rose Herbs
https://mountainroseherbs.com

JUST FOR FUN

This song, **Dandelion**, is by my partner, BethyLoveLight.
https://youtu.be/ojLAH-dkDvE

REFERENCES

Attenborough, David. *The Private Life of Plants*. Princeton, NJ: Princeton University Press, 1995.

Barash, Cathy Wilkinson. *Edible Flowers*. Golden, CO: Fulcrum Publishing, 1993.

Barnett, Robert. *Tonics*. New York: HarperCollins, 1997.

Bensky, Dan, Andrew Gamble, and Ted Kaptchuk. *Chinese Herbal Medicine: Materia Medica*. Seattle: Eastland Press, 1986.

Bremness, Lesley. *The Complete Book of Herbs*. New York: Viking Studio Books, 1988.

Brown, O. Phelps. *The Complete Herbalist*. Van Nuys, CA: Newcastle Publishing, 1993.

Castleman, Michael. *The Healing Herbs*. Emmaus, PA: Rodale Press, 1991.

Chevallier, Andrew. *The Encyclopedia of Medicinal Plants*. New York: DK Publishing, 1996.

Cunningham, Donna. *Flower Remedies Handbook*. New York: Sterling Publishing Co., 1992.

D'Amelio, Frank. *The Botanical Practitioner*. Bellmore, NY: Holistic Publishing, 1982.

Dawson, Adele G. *Herbs: Partners in Life*. Rochester, VT: Healing Arts Press, 1991.

Dobelis, Inge N., ed. *Magic and Medicine of Plants*. Pleasantville, NY: Reader's Digest Association, 1986.

Duke, James A. *The Green Pharmacy*. Emmaus, PA: Rodale Books, 1997.

Faber, K. "The Dandelion *Taraxacum officinale*." *Die Pharmazie* 13:423–36, 1958.

Felter, Harvey Wickes, and John Uri Lloyd. *King's American Dispensatory*. Portland, OR: Eclectic Medical Publications, 1983.

Fielder, Mildred. *Plant Medicine and Folklore*. New York: Winchester Press, 1975.

Frawley, David, and Vasant Lad. *The Yoga of Herbs*. Santa Fe, NM: Lotus Press, 1986.

Gail, Peter A. *The Dandelion Celebration*. Cleveland, OH: Goosefoot Acres, 1994.

Grieve, Margaret. *A Modern Herbal*. New York: Dover Publications, 1971.

Harvey, Clare G., and Amanda Cochrane. *The Encyclopaedia of Flower Remedies*. San Francisco: Thorsons, 1995.

Heinerman, John. *Heinerman's Encyclopedia of Healing Herbs & Spices*. West Nyack, NY: Parker Publishing, 1996.

———. *Heinerman's Encyclopedia of Healing Juices*. Englewood Cliffs, NJ: Prentice Hall, 1994.

———. *Scientific Validation of Herbal Medicine*. Orem, UT: Bi-World Publishers, 1979.

Hobbs, Christopher. "*Taraxacum officinale*: A Monograph and Literature Review." *Eclectic Dispensatory*. Portland, OR: Eclectic Medical Publications, 1989.

Hoffmann, David. *The Holistic Herbal*. Findhorn, Scotland: The Findhorn Press, 1983.

Jones, Pamela. *Just Weeds*. New York: Prentice-Hall Press, 1991.

Keville, Kathi. *The Illustrated Herb Encyclopedia*. New York: Mallard Press, 1991.

Kirschmann, Gayla, and John D. Kirschmann. *Nutrition Almanac*. San Francisco: McGraw Hill, 1996.

Kotobuki Seiyaku, K. K. Pat. *Japanese Pharmacopoeia* 81/10117 (1981), Japan.

Kroeber, L. "Pharmacology and Therapeutic Use of Inulin Preparations." *Die Pharmazie* 5:122–27, 1950.

Lowenfeld, Claire, and Philippa Back. *The Complete Book of Herbs and Spices*. Boston: Little Brown and Company, 1974.

Mabey, Richard. *The New Age Herbalist*. New York: Collier Books, 1988.

McIntyre, Anne. *Flower Power*. New York: Henry Holt and Company, 1996.

McVicar, Jekka. *Herbs for the Home*. New York: Viking Studio Books, 1994.

Meyer, Clarence. *The Herbalist Almanac*. Glenwood, IL: Meyerbooks, 1977.

Mills, Simon Y. *The Essential Book of Herbal Medicine*. New York: Penguin Group, 1991.

Mills, Simon, and Steven Finando. *Alternatives in Healing*. New York: New American Library, 1988.

Mowrey, Daniel B. *Herbal Tonic Therapies*. New Canaan, CT: Keats Publishing, 1993.

Murray, Michael T. *The Healing Power of Herbs*. Rocklin, CA: Prima Publishing, 1995.

Null, Gary. *Herbs for the Seventies*. New York: Dell Books 1972.

Ody, Penelope. *The Complete Medicinal Herbal*. New York: DK Publishing, 1993.

———. *Home Herbal*. New York: DK Publishing, 1995.

Pahlow, Mannfried. *Healing Plants*. Hauppauge, NY: Barron's Publishing, 1993.

Phillips, Roger, and Nicky Foy. *The Random House Book of Herbs*. New York: Random House, 1990.

Rácz-Kotilla, E., G. Rácz, and A. Solomon. "The Action of *Taraxacum officinale* Extracts on the Body Weight and Diuresis of Laboratory Animals." *Planta Medica* 26:212–17, 1974.

St. Claire, Debra. *The Herbal Medicine Cabinet*. Berkeley, CA: Celestial Arts, 1997.

Sanders, Jack. *Hedgemaids and Fairy Candles*. Camden, ME: Ragged Mountain Press, 1993.

Scully, Virginia. *A Treasury of American Indian Herbs*. New York: Crown Publishers, 1972.

Stuart, Malcolm. *The Encyclopedia of Herbs and Herbalism*. New York: Crescent Books, 1979.

Treben, Maria. *Health Through God's Pharmacy*. Steyer, Austria: Wilhelm Ennsthaler, 1984.

Weed, Susun. *Breast Cancer? Breast Health!* Woodstock, New York: Ash Tree Publishing, 1996.

———. *Healing Wise*. Woodstock, New York: Ash Tree Publishing, 1989.

Weiner, Michael. *Weiner's Herbal*. Mill Valley, CA: Quantum Books, 1990.

Weiner, Michael, and Janet Weiner. *Herbs That Heal*. Mill Valley, CA: Quantum Books, 1994.

Wheelwright, Edith Grey. *Medicinal Plants and Their History*. New York: Dover Publications, 1974.

Willard, Terry. *A Textbook of Modern Herbology*. Calgary, Canada: Progressive Publishing, 1988.

———. *The Wild Rose Scientific Herbal*. Calgary, Canada: College of Natural Healing, 1991.

Wood, Magda Ironside. *Herbs*. Secaucus, NJ: Castle Books, 1975.

INDEX

189

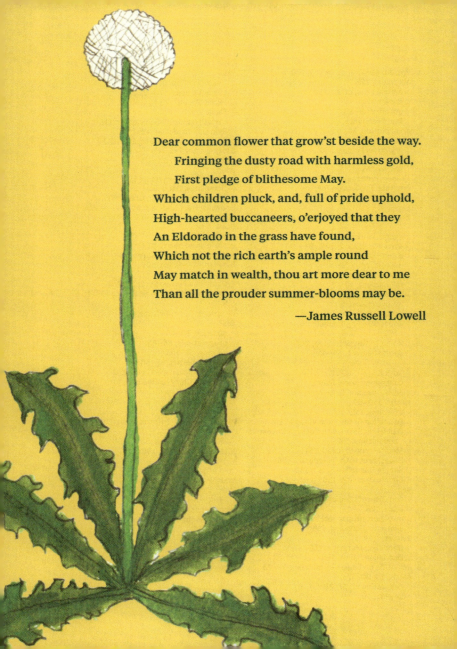

Dear common flower that grow'st beside the way.
   Fringing the dusty road with harmless gold,
   First pledge of blithesome May.
Which children pluck, and, full of pride uphold,
High-hearted buccaneers, o'erjoyed that they
An Eldorado in the grass have found,
Which not the rich earth's ample round
May match in wealth, thou art more dear to me
Than all the prouder summer-blooms may be.

—James Russell Lowell